T0374955

From Skepticism to Competence

ETHNOGRAPHIC ENCOUNTERS AND DISCOVERIES
A series edited by Stefan Timmermans

From Skepticism to Competence

How American Psychiatrists Learn Psychotherapy

MARIANA CRACIUN

The University of Chicago Press   Chicago and London

The University of Chicago Press, Chicago 60637
The University of Chicago Press, Ltd., London
© 2024 by The University of Chicago
Published 2024
Printed in the United States of America

33 32 31 30 29 28 27 26 25 24   1 2 3 4 5

ISBN-13: 978-0-226-83389-7 (cloth)
ISBN-13: 978-0-226-83391-0 (paper)
ISBN-13: 978-0-226-83390-3 (e-book)
DOI: https://doi.org/10.7208/chicago/9780226833903.001.0001

Library of Congress Cataloging-in-Publication Data

Names: Craciun, Mariana, author.
Title: From skepticism to competence : how American psychiatrists learn
    psychotherapy / Mariana Craciun.
Other titles: How American psychiatrists learn psychotherapy | Ethnographic
    encounters and discoveries.
Description: Chicago : The University of Chicago Press, 2024. | Series:
    Ethnographic encounters and discoveries | Includes bibliographical
    references and index.
Identifiers: LCCN 2023042115 | ISBN 9780226833897 (cloth) |
    ISBN 9780226833910 (paperback) | ISBN 9780226833903 (ebook)
Subjects: LCSH: Psychotherapy—Study and teaching—United States. |
    Psychiatry—Study and teaching—United States. | Psychiatrists—
    Education—United States. | Medical education—United States.
Classification: LCC RC459.5.U6 C73 2024 | DDC 616.89/140076—dc23/
    eng/20231103
LC record available at https://lccn.loc.gov/2023042115

CONTENTS

PREFACE

By many accounts, psychiatry is facing a crisis. Over more than four decades, the profession has committed the bulk of its resources and time to tracing the roots of mental illnesses in the brain. This shift has transformed the profession's identity and our collective understanding of mental illness. But many argue that the scientific and treatment benefits have been meager. Psychiatrists have yet to offer a definitive explanation for what causes mental illnesses. There are drugs that work for some patients, but they are not much better than those discovered decades ago. The classification and diagnosis of mental illnesses has proven to be, according to prominent members of the profession, a failed project. All the while, psychiatry is increasingly faulted for having grown so preoccupied with the brain that it has lost sight of the mind. The picture that emerges is one of a profession ill equipped to help its patients.

This is particularly troublesome at a time when Americans' mental health is itself facing a crisis, as more and younger people are diagnosed with depression and anxiety and are dying by suicide. Increasingly, mental health professionals and their work are coming under the microscope. Contemporary psychiatrists appear caught up in a biological web woven partly by their own profession, partly by insurance and pharmaceutical companies, and partly by patients themselves. The common image is that of the harried physician who, for reasons of time, money, and professional training, assesses patients' symptoms, assigns diagnoses, and prescribes psychiatric medications, frequently in ten minutes or less.

This picture is not wrong, but it is incomplete. Though much of their training and practice is dedicated to pharmacology, psychiatrists do learn more than how to prescribe. In fact, to become credentialed, they must also develop competence in psychotherapy, a combination of talk and behavioral interventions. Psychotherapy helps psychiatrists develop new ways of talking with their patients, conceiving of their problems, and formulating solutions. But we know little about how psychiatrists themselves deal with the demands of learning a radically distinct way to doctor.

Psychotherapy training encapsulates psychiatry's predicament, split between being a medical specialty that tends to the diseased body and a professional mission that centers on caring for patients' inner lives. For its apprentices, it can trigger an identity crisis, raising fundamental questions about what it means to be a doctor. Drawing on observations in a psychiatry training program, this book follows a group of residents as they struggle to reconcile competing visions of mental illness and its treatment, whether biological or psychotherapeutic. The residents come to psychotherapy with the skepticism of pharmacologists, reflecting their field's commitment to the brain and its functioning. But, through interactions with colleagues and instructors, they gradually come to view psychotherapy as a coherent and legitimate set of treatments that merit their own place in their professional tool kit. The residents' experiences reflect the challenges of a broader shift in medical training away from a singular focus on scientific knowledge and toward an emphasis on patient care. They also suggest that psychiatry already has within its repertoire one solution to the dual crises facing it and its patients: when drugs are not enough, talking and listening can help.

1 * Learning to Doctor in Psychiatry

Roy Grinker, a leading figure in the field of psychiatry, spoke to a group of colleagues in 1964 about the fate of their profession. He described psychoanalysis, the dominant approach at the time, as "mired in a theoretical rut vigilantly guarded by the orthodox." "Prevented from commingling with science," Grinker stressed, psychoanalysis had failed to "become the therapeutic answer."[1] Grinker's views, in the minority at the time, would become widely shared as psychiatry shifted its attention toward the brain and pharmacological treatments. Three decades later, psychiatrist Robert Klitzman recalled a medical school classmate telling him dismissively that the specialization was "just beginning to move away from witchcraft, slowly modernizing with the introduction of more effective drugs and more scientific approaches."[2] The psychiatry of the 1980s was, in other words, finally leaving behind psychoanalytic witchcraft and joining the rest of medicine through its commitment to science. Closer to the contemporary moment, Jeffrey Lieberman, the former president of the American Psychiatric Association, published a book in 2015 in which he described psychoanalysis as "a plague upon American medicine, infecting every institution of psychiatry with its dogmatic and antiscientific mind-set."[3] In contrast, he deemed twenty-first-century psychiatry the "medicine of the brain" and distinguished it from its talk therapeutic precursor because it "can offer scientific, humane, and *effective* treatments to those suffering from mental illness."[4] Such treatments, Lieberman made clear, revolve around psychiatric drugs.

This narrative of progress from the "dark ages" of psychoanalysis to the enlightened practice of contemporary biological psychiatry has also shaped psychiatrists' views of other forms of psychotherapy.[5] Since the early 1980s, treatments of mental illness that revolve around talk and behavioral interventions have proliferated, gaining increased visibility and legitimacy. Psychodynamic psychotherapy, derived from psychoanalysis, remains widely practiced, though less so by psychiatrists themselves.

Other therapies, such as cognitive behavioral therapy (CBT), dialectical behavioral therapy (DBT), and interpersonal psychotherapy (IPT) have risen to prominence as well. Psychiatrists remain unconvinced. According to Thomas Insel, former director of the National Institute of Mental Health (NIMH), psychodynamic psychotherapy is about as useful as "talking with an empathic friend or pastor," far from other "powerful, scientifically proven treatments" available today. And while he counts among the latter not only medications but also psychotherapies such as CBT, he decries the staying power of the psychodynamic approach, attributing it to a lack of quality control and oversight among psychotherapists.[6] Finally, even as Insel and others praise CBT and related therapies for being "evidence-based," they nevertheless view them as secondary to psychiatric drugs and relegate them to the domain of psychologists and social workers.[7] As one psychiatrist put it, CBT has been "standardized and manualized," which means that "any reasonably intelligent, well-motivated 'generic therapist'" can "administer" it.[8] Whether because it is unscientific or because it is it is too mechanical and straightforward, psychotherapy is simply not for psychiatrists.

*

It is within this larger context that I arrived at Shorewood to join the psychiatry residents as they were learning psychotherapy.[9] During one of the initial meetings of the rotation in dialectical behavioral therapy—a set of cognitive and behavioral interventions for patients who have considered suicide or been diagnosed with borderline personality disorder[10]—Nora, the experienced social worker who led the DBT group, asked the seven residents in attendance a hypothetical question: "So you prescribe a certain medication for your patient and they refuse to take it. How are you going to be effective with that patient?" Alex, a resident early in the fourth postgraduate year (PGY-4), jumped in: "Up the dose!"[11] Laughter erupted around the room. Though at the time I viewed Alex's humor as his implicit acknowledgment of the routine dilemmas of psychiatric doctoring, I later understood it in a different light.

As he dug in his heels against the imaginary patient, the resident retreated into what he knew, into biological psychiatry, implicitly rejecting the therapy-specific strategies Nora was primed to offer. Alex anticipated a shift in epistemic and professional frame and positioned himself against it. His reaction was not entirely surprising. The residents had spent the first two years of their training mastering medication treatments in the hospital. They continued to work as psychopharmacologists, prescribing psychiatric medications, when they transitioned to the clinic in their third postgraduate year (PGY-3). Yet this same transition also signaled the beginning of their psychotherapy training. The shift did not come easy. As they learned talk and behavioral treatments, the junior psychiatrists had to inhabit roles that were epistemically distinct and professionally challenging. They met these roles with skepticism.

Nevertheless, months later, in a cognitive behavioral therapy meeting, I heard Alex offer a different perspective. He told his colleagues that he uses CBT as he talks "to patients about what they're experiencing." "I had a girl come in saying that she's really depressed and, she was saying, she couldn't see the point of living," Alex explained. "I told her that depression distorts her thoughts, and if we looked objectively at her life, I would find reasons to go on living. It resonated with her to do that. I thought I had to counter that thought that she was having, so I think [CBT] gave me a framework for talking about that." Speaking in typical CBT language— about the patient's "distorted" thoughts, "countering" them, and assessing life "objectively"—Alex showcased his newfound psychotherapeutic skills. His skepticism had abated, giving way to competence.

How do psychiatry residents, firmly rooted in biological approaches, overcome their skepticism and become competent in talk and behavioral approaches? More broadly, how do they come to see the various psychotherapies as legitimate and worthwhile complements and even alternatives to pharmacology? The residents face two related challenges as they begin psychotherapy training. Fundamental differences between biological and psychotherapeutic approaches amount to what I came to think of as *epistemic friction*.[12] In addition, psychotherapy training imposes a role reversal on residents, pegging them as novices just as they are moving toward greater independence. This, in turn, produces *professional friction*: mismatches between their anticipated and their actual roles. Together, epistemic and professional frictions prompt the residents to approach psychotherapy with skepticism. This book tells the story of how, with the support of colleagues, instructors, and supervisors, psychiatry residents manage the epistemic and professional frictions inherent in their roles and successfully expand their professional repertoires, moving from skepticism to competence. But to understand why trainees in contemporary psychiatry find themselves in such contradictory positions to begin with, we must turn to their profession's unsettled history.

The Mind and the Brain in Psychiatry

Despite decades of theorizing and research, psychiatry continues to lack definitive answers to fundamental questions about what causes mental illness, whom it affects and why, and how to best treat it. Historically, the profession has been dominated by what historian Jonathan Sadowsky has described as a "continual tension" between a somatic vision that locates mental illness and its cure in the body and a psychological one that seeks solutions in talk and behavior change.[13] Though these perspectives have coexisted throughout psychiatry's history, their alliance has been, at best, uneasy.

The residents I spent time with at Shorewood in the early 2010s trained in a context defined by psychiatry's turn toward pharmacology and the brain. When psychopharmaceuticals were discovered, accidentally, in the 1950s and '60s, psychoanalysis was ascendant in the US.[14] At the time, the approach offered psychiatry a coherent and compelling system of ideas to make sense of problems ranging from shell shock to schizophrenia.[15] In addition, investments in psychoanalytic training and research by NIMH and the prominent role that psychoanalysts, Karl and William Menninger principal among them, played in reforming the nation's mental health care system boosted its credibility.[16]

By the late 1950s, psychoanalytically trained psychiatrists dominated the profession. Though the 1950s and '60s had their blockbuster drugs, such as Miltown (meprobamate), a widely prescribed minor tranquilizer, psychoanalysts viewed them with ambivalence.[17] Psychotropic medications were secondary to the work of uncovering patients' unconscious conflicts. Residents who were training during this period prepared for a career spent in a private office equipped with a couch on which a relatively small number of typically well-to-do patients could recline several times a week and uncover the roots of their problems through dreamwork and free association.[18] In this context, drugs played merely a supportive role.

But a series of economic, structural, and epistemic changes in the 1970s made this model of practice increasingly untenable. Health insurance companies began to assume a larger role in paying for mental health treatments, while the federal government and individual states withdrew their support for hospital care.[19] At the same time, the move toward deinstitutionalization meant that fewer and sicker patients were cared for in hospitals, while those who could function outside the institution would receive treatment in community centers.[20] For psychiatry residents, this translated into increasingly few opportunities to learn psychoanalysis at their primary training sites; namely, hospitals. Practicing this more time-intensive treatment also became nearly impossible with the rise of managed care in the 1990s, which further shortened hospital stays and abbreviated office visits.[21]

In addition, beginning in the 1970s, a reimagining of psychiatry's epistemic foundation was under way. Some psychiatrists were becoming increasingly interested in better understanding the causes, manifestations, and scope of mental illnesses, and doing so outside a psychoanalytic framework. This interest crystallized in a focus on diagnosis, especially as it was codified in the *Diagnostic and Statistical Manual of Mental Disorders* (known familiarly as the DSM), psychiatry's compendium of diagnoses. The first two editions of the DSM, crafted by psychoanalysts, eschewed the kind of standardization and quantification necessary for conducting large-scale research. But in 1972, a group of psychiatrists from the Washington University in St. Louis published an article in the *Archives of General Psychiatry* delineating a set of principles for identifying fifteen mental disorders.[22] "Diagnosis," they argued, "has functions as important in psychiatry as elsewhere in medicine."[23] To the lead author, John Feighner, and his colleagues, the elaboration of diagnoses that can be arrived at on the basis of observable behaviors would not only make psychiatry scientific but would also bring it into the medical fold.

The group's efforts facilitated two related transformations in the field. First, they culminated in the revision of psychiatry's diagnostic manual and the 1980 publication of the much touted and critiqued DSM-III. This edition emphasized the observable aspects of mental illness, contributing to a larger shift in psychiatric practices away from unconscious conflicts and toward researching and chemically managing brain mechanisms of mental disease.[24] Second, the publication of the Feighner criteria signaled the field's growing discontent with psychoanalysis. Psychoanalysts were largely excluded from the DSM's third revision and, over a few short years in the 1980s, lost their leading positions in psychiatry departments and their roles in the American Psychiatric Association.[25] In the psychotherapeutic domain, psychoanalysis was also being replaced as the preeminent approach by cognitive therapy (later, CBT) and IPT, both of which gained momentum as researchers demonstrated and publicized their efficacy.[26] Psychoanalysis was increasingly marginalized, viewed as a weakness in a field that sought to establish its scientific bona fides.

Psychiatry's turn to biology in the 1980s reshaped how its practitioners were trained and what they did once they graduated. Unlike earlier cohorts of psychiatrists, most of whom had planned on becoming psychoanalysts in private practice, those training in the 1980s and 1990s were increasingly less likely to follow that path.[27] They were also less likely to learn psychotherapy and more likely to spend their time prescribing medications.[28] Today, a majority of psychiatrists spend their time with patients solely managing medications, and that is the doctoring approach that residents learn. This brain-based vision of mental illness has been widely successful outside the profession as well, having come to define the public imaginary. Most Americans view their suffering as "neurobiological," to echo Joseph Davis, and, as of 2020, 16 percent of US adults took psychiatric medications for their mental health.[29]

Yet just as our collective reliance on such drugs seems to have reached its apex, biological psychiatry has come under increased criticism. Some patients are calling into question the necessity of psychiatric medications, and larger numbers are turning to psychotherapy as their treatment of choice.[30] Psychiatrists themselves are growing more skeptical of neurobiology's early promises, questioning the usefulness of the DSM and the effectiveness of some of the most commonly prescribed psychiatric drugs, and criticizing the "chemical imbalance" theory that has come to define the public's understanding of mental illness.[31]

For psychiatry residents, these challenges are not simply abstract matters. In fact, becoming an expert psychiatrist is, nowadays, as much about learning to prescribe as it is about understanding the limitations and drawbacks of pharmacological treatments. Though their day-to-day work continues to revolve around learning about and prescribing medications, psychiatry residents frequently come up against the limits of their chemical tools. Patients cannot or do not take their psychiatric medications and, frequently enough, do not get better when they do. Psychotherapy can help psychiatrists care for their patients, but only if these clinicians overcome their long-standing skepticism against nonpharmacological approaches. Since the beginning of the twenty-first century, changes in accreditation standards have compelled psychiatrists to face their doubts.

Psychotherapy in Psychiatry

Writing in the pages of *Academic Psychiatry*, Lisa Mellman and Jeremy Beresin, two psychiatrists involved in graduate education at Columbia University and Harvard University, respectively, attributed the erosion of therapeutic training to a confluence of factors.[32] Some had to do with the economics of care, including the rapid shrinkage of hospital stays that drastically curtailed opportunities for residents to work with patients over the long term. Additionally, they pointed to accreditation standards or, rather, a lack of specific requirements and uniform guidelines for what to teach, as bearing some responsibility for this shift.[33] Another factor is also worth mentioning here: psychiatry's struggle to establish its place in medicine. The specialty's enduring liminality, exacerbated by its epistemic uncertainties, shaped its educational priorities. Its turn to biology in the early 1980s seemed to offer it an indispensable hook for joining the rest of medicine.

Whatever its causes, the field's shift away from psychotherapy was swiftly felt. Psychiatrists Sheldon Miller and Daniel Winstead, both of whom figured prominently in setting accreditation standards around the turn of the twenty-first century, joined by James Scully Jr., the medical director of the American Psychiatric Association during the same period, recounted that "concern over an apparent atrophy of psychotherapy skills among recent graduates" was "widespread."[34] Whereas the residents knew pharmacology, they did not understand "that symptoms may have arisen in the context of life events or relationships which have particular meanings to the patient."[35] "Additionally," Miller and his coauthors pointed out, "there was a perception voiced by many examiners on the American Board of Psychiatry and Neurology (ABPN) Part II oral exam"—the ABPN being the body responsible for certification—"that too many candidates were unable to conduct an empathic interview."[36] Without psychotherapy, psychiatry residents did not know how to talk with their patients nor understood why they suffered.

Calls for reintroducing psychotherapy into psychiatry's educational curriculum grew more insistent during the 1990s, but they reflected psychiatry's biological commitments. "The goal is no longer to teach all residents how to practice psychoanalytic psychotherapy," a group of psychiatrists argued in the pages of the *American Journal of Psychiatry* as early as 1990.[37] Rather, "the goal is to turn out psychodynamically informed and sophisticated psychiatrists" who would be equipped to understand and treat their patients with medications.[38] They would also be better prepared to supervise other professionals in the field, such as psychologists and social workers, who are likely the providers of psychotherapy. "At stake" in debates about what residents ought to learn, the authors wrote, "is our vision of the future psychiatrist."[39] That vision, at least according to these physicians, had to include not simply pharmacology and the emerging field of neuroscience but also psychotherapy.

It would take another decade to put that vision into practice. As discontent around psychiatric education grew, proponents of psychotherapy training found an unlikely opening in the late 1990s. Nationally, the Accreditation Council for Graduate Medical Education (ACGME), a nonprofit organization responsible for accrediting all medical specialties, announced a transition to an "outcome based competency model" which would assess the aptitudes of all residents, regardless of specialty, in "patient care, medical knowledge, practice-based learning and improvement, interpersonal and communication skills, professionalism, and systems-based practice."[40] As the field of medicine began to emphasize "patient care" and "interpersonal and communication skills," psychiatrists were primed to rediscover the value of psychotherapy.

In advance of the national change, the Residency Review Committee (RRC) for psychiatry, a subgroup of the ACGME, resolved to mandate evidence of competence in five therapeutic approaches: brief psychotherapy, cognitive behavioral therapy, combined psychotherapy and pharmacotherapy, psychodynamic therapy, and supportive therapy.[41] This requirement, to be implemented in 2001 following the broader ACGME shift, was deemed daunting by some residency directors, particularly those in relatively underresourced programs. Others were concerned with how the residents' psychotherapeutic skills could be assessed. "In contrast to the summative competency definitions for procedural competencies used in other parts of medicine," a group of psychiatrists pointed out in 2003, "psychotherapy competencies are not so cut-and-dried, nor are they so readily observed."[42] In psychotherapy, there was no equivalent of doing "a great job of removing an appendix from start to finish."[43] Psychotherapeutic skills were more intangible and harder to pinpoint. They were thus more challenging to teach and assess.

But the requirements also rekindled debates about the place of psychoanalysis, and more specifically its offspring, psychodynamic psychotherapy, in psychiatry.[44] Tensions were especially pronounced during a 2001 exchange between Psychiatry RRC chair Dr. Daniel Winstead and NIMH director Dr. Steven Hyman.[45] Hyman objected that, saddled with new psychotherapy requirements, psychiatry residencies left little time for trainees to do research and help cement psychiatry's scientific base. Although "we would all agree that psychotherapy is absolutely critical," the NIMH director argued, the RRC's inclusion of psychodynamic psychotherapy was ill-conceived. In fact, Hyman stressed, "I think we have to, as a field, grapple with what it means that you [the psychiatry RRC] have succumbed to historical and collegial pressures and have put up as a requirement something that is not evidence-based and for which the practitioners are not even, by NIMH applications standards, interested in being in the game." The "game" was that of conducting and implementing efficacy research akin to other medical subfields. For the head of the NIMH, psychodynamic psychiatrists did not merit a seat at the training table.

Nevertheless, historical precedent held. When I began my fieldwork in late 2009, ACGME standards required that psychiatry residents be trained in patient care that included "applying supportive, psychodynamic, and cognitive-behavioral psychotherapies to both brief and long-term individual practice."[46] In addition, they called for "exposure to family, couples, group and other individual evidence-based psychotherapies."[47] In 2013, a shift in how medical specialties get accredited led to renewed emphasis on psychotherapeutic skills in psychiatry—skills that are now assessed with a system of "milestones."[48]

Contemporary requirements include expected facilities with diagnosis and pharmacological treatment and an understanding of the epidemiology of mental illnesses and of a range of neurologic disorders. But one of the first requirements is that residents "demonstrate competence" in "forging a therapeutic alliance" with patients of various backgrounds.[49]

Today, novice psychiatrists are expected to learn the "central theoretical principles across the three core psychotherapeutic modalities: supportive, psychodynamic, [and] cognitive-behavioral," and be able to summarize "the evidence base" for each.[50] Furthermore, they must ably analyze "the evidence base for combining psychotherapy and pharmacotherapy."[51] Practically, a skilled resident-therapist "identifies and reflects the core feelings, key issues and what the issues mean to the patients during the session, while managing the emotional content and feelings elicited" and, at an even higher level of mastery, connects "feelings, recurrent/central themes/schemas and their meaning to the patient as they shift within and across sessions."[52] Such abilities depend on a sustained engagement with the theories and practices of psychodynamic and cognitive behavioral therapies.

Shorewood residents, trained three years before the "milestone" framework was implemented and ten years before their most recent revision, were already ahead of the curve. Along with abundant avenues for honing their biological expertise, the program also offered them opportunities to develop their psychotherapeutic know-how. Nevertheless, as organizational and policy scholars have long shown, there is a difference between creating a requirement, setting up the structures necessary for implementing it, and discovering what implementation looks like in practice.[53] For the residents, becoming competent in therapeutic modalities—alongside biopsychiatry—meant stepping into doctoring roles organized around radically different assumptions about mental illness and its treatment. I outline each of these next.

Ways to Doctor

The ACGME requires training programs to equip psychiatry residents with competence in biopsychiatry and psychotherapy, specifically psychodynamic and cognitive behavioral approaches. In keeping with psychiatry's current biological focus, the vast majority of its residents' training is taken up by the pharmacological management of patients' symptoms. Psychiatry residents enter the specialization after four years of medical school focused largely on the biological dimensions of disease. They then spend their first two postgraduate years—the internship year (PGY-1) and the first year of psychiatric training (PGY-2)—working primarily with hospitalized patients whose acute conditions and short stays require immediate intervention. Learning psychiatry in this context compels the residents, as anthropologist T. M. Luhrmann explained, to think of mental illness "as an organic disease, a 'thing' underlying and generating the symptoms."[54] And treating such disease means learning how to diagnose it and address its symptoms with medications.[55] Writing medication prescriptions carries particular symbolic power for psychiatrists, especially those earlier in their training. Pharmacology, Luhrmann writes, "makes young residents feel like doctors" because "they are doing something to relieve the body's pain."[56]

Psychodynamic therapy challenges psychiatry residents to learn a completely different way to doctor. The approach evolved from psychoanalysis, a treatment formulated by Sigmund Freud in the early twentieth century.[57] Unlike its better-known (and critiqued) predecessor, psychodynamic psychotherapy does not necessitate the use of a couch, nor the high frequency of weekly sessions focused on dreamwork and free association. Despite such practical differences, the approach does share with psychoanalysis a commitment to understanding patients' unconscious conflicts and their manifestations in relationships. In a widely used "basic text" for residents, psychiatrist and psychoanalyst Glen Gabbard advises that "symptoms and behaviors [. . .] are determined by complex and often unconscious forces."[58] To understand such forces, a psychodynamic therapist relies on "the patient's transference" as well as their own "countertransference." *Transference* is a psychoanalytic term used to describe how we unconsciously endow present experiences and relationships with feelings and expectations from the past.[59] Unraveling the workings and meanings of patients' transference while being mindful of their own feelings and reactions, known as *countertransference*, is the psychodynamic therapist's principal goal. Psychodynamic psychotherapy, Gabbard asserts, helps patients achieve "a sense of authenticity and uniqueness."[60]

To practice this approach, the residents must learn new ways to think about mental illness and go about its treatment. Even though they may still be prescribing medications for the patients they treat psychodynamically, they have to also become adept at eliciting and understanding the patients' life stories along with tracking their symptoms. They must move beyond empathy and develop new ways to interpret their patients' and their own inner lives. They have to think about the nuances of the therapeutic relationship, treating it not simply as a conduit for assuring patients' adherence to treatment but as a magnifying glass for their unconscious conflicts. Finally, patience rather than action must become the residents' principal stance. Used to deploying their know-how by writing a prescription, the residents must accustom themselves to listening more and saying less, to guiding rather than telling.

Cognitive behavioral therapy offers psychiatry residents a more familiar model of doctoring. Aaron Beck, a psychiatrist, elaborated cognitive therapy, CBT's precursor, in the 1960s under the influence of psychoanalytic ideas. But his approach departs from psychodynamic psychotherapy in radical ways. Beck borrowed from cognitive science the theory that people orient themselves in the world by relying on *schemas*, mental models that help them make sense of their social environment and their own place in it.[61] People who suffer from depression, Beck argued, tend to have overwhelmingly negative schemas about their self-worth, their "characteristics," and their "performance."[62] The thoughts that make up such schemas come up automatically and are taken for granted—they are believed without questioning. They also fuel the negative feelings associated with depression. Most important, unlike the unconscious desires and motivations that needed to be unearthed through psychoanalysis, such thoughts are readily available for patients and their therapists to investigate and modify. Consequently, cognitive therapists are tasked "with the identification, appraisal, and correction of the specific idiosyncratic depressive cognitions" that drive patients' ill feelings.[63] After cognitive therapy joined forces with behaviorism to form CBT, the modification of behavior became as essential as changing distorted thoughts.[64]

With CBT, the residents find themselves on more recognizable ground. Here, they can continue to rely on the DSM to identify and classify patients' symptoms. And, just as they would in a psychopharmacology appointment, they make use of scales, such as the Beck Depression Inventory and the corresponding scale for anxiety, the Hamilton Depression Scale, or the Patient Health Questionnaire, to measure and track patients' problems. Moreover, akin to pharmacology where they write prescriptions, in CBT they can also "give" patients something, as one of the residents put it. Typically, this offering includes a list, such as the "automatic thoughts checklist," or a form, such as the "thought record" or the "activity schedule." Much like taking their medications on a regular basis, patients in CBT are expected to complete "homework" based on these worksheets. In this approach, the residents' principal challenge is learning to think beyond symptoms to disentangle patients' configurations of thoughts, feelings, and behaviors while judiciously choosing targets of cognitive or behavioral modification. Nevertheless, CBT, like biopsychiatry, affords residents an authoritative role as they instruct patients on the nature of their suffering and the means to lessen it.

In having to learn these distinct doctoring approaches, the residents must move between "epistemic cultures," to borrow science and technology scholar Karin Knorr Cetina's term.[65] Biological psychiatry, psychodynamic psychotherapy, and CBT have their own "arrangements and mechanisms"—social, technical, empirical, ideational—by which they construct legitimate knowledge about mental illness. As they learn each approach, psychiatry residents confront significant disjunctures on basic questions about how symptoms should be interpreted, whether mental illness is a disease of the brain, a problem of relationships, or one of disordered thoughts and behaviors, and whether it is best treated chemically, relationally, or cognitively and behaviorally. Friction is built into the experience of working across epistemic boundaries, and skepticism its inevitable effect.

The Conundrums of Becoming a Professional

Three social scientific perspectives can help us make sense of the residents' challenges: scholarship on professional socialization, research on professional identities and work tasks, and writing on contradictory roles. I address each in turn.

PROFESSIONAL SOCIALIZATION

Much of what we know about professional socialization has centered on the transformation of beginners into experts. A simplified version of the typical narrative looks like this: Novices enter a professional "epistemic community" as students or trainees.[66] After going through a variety of rituals and learning how to navigate the epistemic community's particular sources of uncertainty, they adopt not only its knowledge and embodied practices but also its norms and its way of thinking about and interacting with the world.[67] Neophytes become professional experts as they are immersed in the culture of their chosen field. Transformed by the process, they come to think, behave, and feel in new, professionally inflected ways.

These accounts, whether in medicine, law, policing, banking and finance, engineering, or air traffic control, are premised on a view of professions and occupations as relatively coherent systems of epistemic practices and cultural beliefs.[68] Partly because of this assumed coherence, the transition from novice to professional is depicted as taking place in a relatively linear fashion. Outsiders gradually become insiders, accumulating professional status with each successful transition, converted into experts where before they were ignorant.[69]

Psychiatry challenges us to reassess this perspective. Long split among different factions, it compels its trainees to move between expertise and relative ignorance, between professional autonomy and subordination. Whether they have to navigate fundamental differences separating various epistemic models of mental illness or negotiate the challenges of being at once professionals and novices, psychiatry residents' experiences are not linear. As trainees, they do not undergo a stepwise progression from student to professional. Instead, they move between these poles at various stages in the program. Nor is the residents' socialization straightforwardly transformative. By the end of their training, their commitment to chemical treatments softens, but, with very few exceptions, psychiatry residents do not become psychotherapists once they graduate.

How do we make sense of the experiences of professionals who are compelled to develop competence in roles and practices that are not simply new but that also contradict their existing assumptions? The psychiatry residents whose stories animate this book struggled with more than the novice uncertainty that has defined studies of socialization since Renee Fox's landmark research on this topic.[70] They also had to confront the epistemic and professional frictions that result from navigating discordant new expectations about doctoring and its practices. And what happens when these professional novices face such demands not as eager neophytes but rather as skeptical observers, reluctant to engage in the process of socialization? We might explain such appeals to skepticism in professional settings as efforts to maintain a valued professional identity in the face of threat, and I turn to this perspective next.

PROFESSIONAL IDENTITY AND CONTROL OVER CORE TASKS

Professionals point to their core tasks to describe what they do and assert who they are.[71] Indeed, the ongoing process of delimiting and safeguarding what they do is the sine qua non of professional groups' existence. Social scientists have shown that such groups must continually defend their domains of knowledge and practice, since their boundaries are, as Andrew Abbott argued, "perpetually in dispute."[72] Whether professionals see such domains, also known as jurisdictions, threatened by competitors or undermined by reforms, they are persistently striving to retain control over tasks that are in line with their valued identities.[73]

Psychiatrists, Owen Whooley has argued, have periodically struggled to reinvent themselves and their core work, partly because of the obstinate "ignorance" that has dogged their attempts to grasp and cure mental illness.[74] Since the mid-twentieth century, such reinvention has largely sought to distance psychiatry from psychotherapy, particularly psychoanalysis, and to privilege the biological study and management of mental illness. In the process, psychiatrists have ceded control over psychotherapy to psychologists and social workers. In a context where biologization seemed to offer the profession a ticket to legitimacy as a medical specialty, this was not particularly problematic. Indeed, psychiatrists' rejection of psychoanalysis, combined with their commitment to pharmacology, has constituted the profession's strategy for maintaining dominance in the broader field of mental health over more than forty years.

But psychotherapy has not entirely disappeared from psychiatry, remaining a competency enshrined in ACGME requirements. As psychiatrists have come to define their professional identities around the chemical management of mental illness, psychotherapy's endurance raises two fundamental questions for the profession: what is psychiatry and what are its core practices? Through this lens, the residents' skepticism can be viewed as a reflection of their profession's own struggles to define itself and its core jurisdiction. Put another way, expressions of doubt are part of the practical work required to maintain a coherent professional identity by drawing boundaries around what is and, more important, what is not, proper psychiatric domain. By deeming psychotherapy the territory of psychologists and social workers, psychiatrists signal their commitment to the more valued identity of medical doctors who, more than simply talking and listening to patients, also treat their illnesses with medications.[75] Alex's joke in the DBT rotation can thus be viewed as part of the symbolic work that psychiatrists perform to maintain their valued roles as pharmacologists, while also subtly enforcing the division of labor in the field.

This perspective would not be wrong. But it would be incomplete. While the residents were invested in upholding biopsychiatry's domain and identity as a medical specialty, this was not their primary concern. Indeed, their more immediate preoccupation was to establish their *own* worth in conditions that seemed geared toward undermining it through contradictory demands. And, if we focused exclusively on the residents' commitments to a biological framework, how would we explain their diminished skepticism and evolving psychotherapeutic competence? Finally, how would we make sense of their expanded doctoring repertoires and the subsequent inflections in their biopsychiatric identities? For potential answers to these questions, we can appeal to the literature on contradictory role demands.

CONTRADICTORY ROLES

The residents' positions in psychotherapy training can be described as "structurally ambivalent," to borrow Robert Merton's and Elinor Barber's concept, organized around "incompatible normative expectations of attitudes, beliefs, and behavior."[76] Sociologists have shown such contradictions to be commonplace in social life, as when people ascribe to divergent cultural values or epistemic norms and practices, or when they move between social statuses or migrate between countries.[77] Merton and Barber stressed that social actors seek to resolve the contradictions in their roles by "blending" divergent expectations "into a functionally consistent whole."[78] From this perspective, the residents' expanding doctoring repertoires and their competence in psychotherapeutic interventions are functional accommodations to program requirements. But this view overlooks the practical work that social actors engage in to overcome contradictions embedded in the process. It also prioritizes the fit between institutional imperatives and identity change, missing potential or partial misalignments.

Indeed, scholars of organizations have argued that professionals are less invested in their organizational identities, for example as employees of a particular hospital or law firm, than they are in their identities as experts with control over particular work tasks.[79] Subsequently, in contrast to the perspective of functional integration, contemporary research has shown that rather than blend incompatible expectations, social actors prioritize some values or norms over others, even in contexts that seem to give them little choice. For professionals, maintaining social status and the integrity of their epistemic and professional identities takes precedence over policy or organizational demands that would undermine these concerns.[80] From this perspective, the residents' skepticism toward psychotherapy can be viewed as a mechanism for maintaining their status by distancing themselves from lower-prestige work. But this would only account for skepticism's defensive function, overlooking the possibilities for change it can enable in the right socioinstitutional contexts.

Skepticism itself has received scant conceptual attention in research on contradictory roles. Whether treated as the implicit counterpoint to religious belief or trust, or as a symbol of political and cultural division,[81] we know less about skepticism's productive possibilities, particularly in epistemic communities that are, as Robert Merton asserted, organized around the management of doubt.[82] Philosopher Isabelle Stengers has argued that skepticism is the "normal response" in scientific exchange, and that the work involved in "conquering" it constitutes both scientific facts and scientists themselves.[83] But what are the practical dimensions of such constitution? How does the work of managing skepticism and constructing valued identities unfold in conditions defined by contradictory demands? Finally, how do we make sense of skepticism's resolution when it does not entail a complete conversion? After all, the residents whose stories are the focus of this book did not renounce biopsychiatry to become psychotherapists. To make sense of their experiences, we need a theory of skepticism that accounts for the contradictions that generate doubt, the contexts that facilitate its collective management, and the conditions that constrain its resolution.

From Skepticism to Competence

The residents' shift from psychotherapy skeptics to competent initiates was not characterized by sudden transformations. Rather, their transition was the result of a cumulative process in which they submitted, sometimes reluctantly, to the demands of being psychotherapy trainees. By the end of their training, the residents developed competence in various psychotherapies along with distinct ways of accommodating their new knowledge into their existing doctoring repertoires. This book tells the story of this process and offers a sociological account of its dynamics; it is a story of skepticism, its collective management, and its resolution.

It is worth reiterating that when I use the term *skepticism*, I am not referring to the kind of misgivings or doubts fostered by the residents' individual histories or personalities, though such factors can moderate whether and how particular trainees take on the part of skeptic during group discussions.[84] To the contrary, far from being an individual characteristic, I propose that skepticism is triggered by role contradictions. Nor should the residents' doubts be confused for the kind of novice uncertainty that is inherent in learning something new. Indeed, the residents were not simply learning new ways to doctor—they were compelled to engage with ideas and practices that contradicted their existing assumptions about doctoring and about themselves. They had to learn to doctor without drugs in a context that had built them up as pharmacologists.

This book starts from the assumption that successful professional socialization entails not only internalizing a particular set of ideas and practices but also, if only implicitly, rejecting others. In other words, professionalization contains within it the makings of skepticism, a potentiality activated by conditions of friction. In turn, skepticism is a stance that enables actors to leverage their existing knowledge and establish their worth and that, in certain contexts, can also foster experimentation with new ideas and tools. Skepticism is inherently unstable—pragmatist philosopher Charles Sanders Peirce described doubt as "an uneasy and dissatisfied state" that spurs people to seek a resolution.[85] When friction is transitory—say, in a hallway interaction with someone whose views are different, or during a short-lived stint with an interdisciplinary team—skepticism remains merely defensive, to borrow Erving Goffman's term, protecting people's existing commitments and identities.[86] In this phase, doubt precludes the kind of epistemic generosity necessary for expanding one's repertoire of action. Yet sustained engagement with new ideas and practices in supportive environments can render skepticism productive. Such environments, the following pages will show, revolve around spaces in which doubts can be shared and addressed by trusted others, where new practices and ideas are opened for observation and discussion, and where low-stakes experimentation can take place.

Early in psychotherapy training, skepticism allowed the residents to claim professional status in the face of novicehood. As they appealed to their biopsychiatric know-how to question psychotherapeutic interventions, they sought to position themselves as more than ignorant novices. But skepticism also afforded them an opening to try out new doctoring approaches partly because it rendered the process of developing therapeutic competence nonthreatening to their budding authority as pharmacologists. Meetings of psychotherapy rotations, with their mix of support, observation, and experimentation, were productive contexts for this process to unfold. As the residents' knowledge of talk and behavioral interventions deepened, skepticism gave way to self-reflexivity. Increasingly aware, they could attend more closely to their doctoring practices and their own subjectivities, as well as their relationships with their patients. Finally, equipped with new knowledge, the residents could approach psychotherapy not as skeptical outsiders but as competent initiates.

Skepticism's resolution should not be taken for the disappearance of professional and epistemic friction. Although the professional contradictions in the residents' roles attenuated as they neared graduation, the epistemic mismatches between biopsychiatry and psychotherapy remain. Moreover, after they graduate, the residents enter a field that, through economic, institutional, and professional arrangements, is set up to maintain divisions between various occupational and epistemic communities. However, skepticism's resolution in psychotherapeutic competence allows the residents to recognize different nonpharmacological approaches as coherent sets of ideas and practices and appeal to them as they deem necessary for patient care. Like learners of a new language, they become conversant enough in psychotherapeutic idioms to deploy them in contextually appropriate ways even as biopsychiatry remains their "native" language.

The Study

Between 2009 and 2011, I spent eighteen months at Shorewood observing how psychiatry residents learned psychotherapy. Their training took place at an outpatient mental health clinic associated with a renowned and well-resourced university system. The clinic is housed in an expansive building that welcomes visitors into an airy atrium where administrative assistants help patients check in for appointments and make payments. A room with armchairs set out in grids forms a spacious waiting area that, I would learn, presented novices with unexpected conundrums when calling up their patients for appointments. Therapy offices, along with conference and training rooms, dot a maze of carpeted, beige, and remarkably quiet hallways. I had to learn my way through the confusingly identical corridors before I could recognize the conference rooms where psychotherapy rotations took place.

My observations focused on group meetings in these rotations, which covered topics ranging from the practical aspects of doing therapy, to psychotherapeutic theories, to discussions of patients and their treatments. Sometimes, the meetings included sessions with patients; on other occasions, experienced psychotherapists came to discuss their own work or that of the residents. Most frequently, meetings started with an instructor inviting the residents to bring up a treatment they needed help with. The volunteer would then deliver a case presentation, which would, in turn, set up the group to offer ideas about treatment. The ensuing discussions were just as much about the theory and practice of psychotherapy as they were about what it means to be a psychotherapist and a biopsychiatrist.

While doing therapy with patients is, without a doubt, a powerful learning experience for the residents, the group discussions they participated in were more productive for my purposes.[87] Their manifest goal was to introduce the residents to the basic assumptions and methods of a particular therapeutic approach and to help them navigate the challenges of implementing these methods. Yet the discussions also extended to the contradictions embedded in the residents' roles, the problems they were facing, and their possible solutions. These meetings revealed how professionals in an unsettled field navigate the conundrums that inevitably emerge at the boundary between particular ways of understanding and treating their object of knowledge, mental illness.

Such conversations were also particularly illuminating of skepticism and its management. The residents were the primary doubters: they questioned the structure of their training, the requirements that they were supposed to meet, the assumptions of certain therapeutic approaches and their relative merits vis-à-vis competing ones, therapy's usefulness for patients, and their supervisors' own methods. For their part, psychotherapy instructors sought to shake the residents' faith in organic treatments of mental illness while also introducing them to the justificatory logics of therapy. They explained why a particular technique worked and how it compared with others. They helped the residents develop mental shortcuts about patients' problems and sought to inspire their confidence in their particular therapeutic approach. In the process, they sought to assuage the residents' skepticism by opening up practical avenues for them to experiment with psychotherapeutic ways of thinking, feeling, and doing.

It is important to point out that although both supervisors and residents did, at times, assert the superiority of their own approach, none aimed to convert the other. Instead, a largely tacit understanding seemed to dominate their exchanges; namely, that they were there to broaden rather than replace the residents' professional tool kit. For the most part, this meant educating the residents so that they can recognize when a patient needs one or another talk therapeutic intervention and be able to make an appropriate referral. Sometimes it meant turning out professionals who could be both biological psychiatrists and psychotherapists.

Book Plan

The following chapters illustrate the residents' struggles with psychotherapy as well as their growing competence in it. The first two chapters detail the fertile ground for skepticism created by the contradictions in the residents' roles. Chapter 2 sets the stage by describing the psychiatric residency and its particular form at Shorewood. Shorewood was ahead of the curve in psychotherapeutic education, offering residents extensive training in psychodynamic and cognitive behavioral approaches, along with interpersonal psychotherapy and couples and marriage therapy. Yet despite these signs of what some in the program called a "balanced" approach to the psychiatric curriculum, the majority of the residents' time was still spent learning and doing pharmacology. This actual imbalance made their transition to psychotherapy ripe for conflict, and the chapter shows the residents trying to negotiate a modicum of professional control through the proxy of time. Chapter 3 offers an account of the frictions the residents faced. Epistemically, they struggled to set aside their earlier reliance on symptoms and the DSM and focus instead on understanding patients' idiosyncratic illness experiences. Differences between biopsychiatric, CBT, and psychodynamic approaches are especially significant, and I show the unique challenges the psychotherapies posed the residents. Professionally, the residents had to contend anew with the dilemmas of supervision, and the chapter shows them navigating their contradictory roles as doctors and novices.

The next three chapters zoom into the residents' skepticism and its management in psychotherapy rotations. I start with the psychotherapy instructors who, as I show in chapter 4, faced an uphill battle seeking to make their approaches legitimate to the biopsychiatrists. To facilitate the residents' practical apprenticeship, the instructors opened the craft of psychotherapy up for observation. Doing so also contributed to legitimating their treatments, and the instructors worked assiduously to enhance the credibility of talk and behavioral approaches to their decidedly biological audience.

Chapters 5 and 6 detail the residents' experiences in CBT and psychodynamic psychotherapy, respectively, showcasing both overlaps and divergences between approaches. In both rotations, the residents' training takes place through case discussions and presentations, and the chapters illuminate their engagement in these rituals of socialization. In chapter 5, I trace the residents' engagement with CBT. Because of its affinities with biopsychiatry, the approach offers them an easier path from skepticism to competence. Unlike in psychodynamic psychotherapy where they must reframe their fundamental assumptions about doctoring, CBT offer them tools and techniques that, akin to psychiatric medications, can be deployed in time-limited contexts. Achieving practical competence in the approach happens partly through role-plays, and I detail the residents' struggles as well as their supports in these pragmatic learning exercises. In chapter 6 I turn to the residents' parallel, if more acute, struggles in psychodynamic training. Unsettled by psychodynamic psychotherapy's focus on patients' inner lives and the dynamics of the therapeutic relationship, the residents approach this training with hesitation and skepticism. But, with time and support from peers and instructors, they become increasingly reflective about the disjunctures between their biopsychiatric doctoring repertoire and the psychodynamic model. Junior residents are encouraged along the path toward competence by their senior colleagues. Their case presentations serve both as models of new ways to doctor and as professional testimonials of psychodynamic psychotherapy's utility.

In the final empirical chapter, I turn my attention to the resolution of skepticism. Chapter 7 finds the residents closer to the end of their psychotherapy training, competently and confidently inhabiting roles as psychotherapy initiates. In CBT, where a sense of practical know-how comes earlier, third- and fourth-year residents showcase their ability to disentangle patients' thoughts, feelings, and behaviors during case discussions and to give able performances in role-plays. In the psychodynamic rotation, the residents competently discuss their patients' and their own inner lives and reflect on the dynamics fueling the therapeutic relationship. The residents diverge, however, in how they integrate these skills with their existing doctoring repertoires, and the chapter ends by describing two alternatives: one in which the residents opt for pragmatic accommodation and another that comes closer to hybrid expertise.

In chapter 8, I offer an integrated theory of the conditions, management, and resolution of professional skepticism. I then provide a reflection on the broader implications of psychotherapy training for psychiatrists, their profession, and the field of mental health at large. Finally, I consider how the conceptual apparatus laid out here might help us better understand professional work and identities, particularly in conditions ripe for friction and skepticism.

2 * Training at Shorewood

Shorewood has a "deserved" reputation of "having a balanced approach to meds and therapy," Dr. Armstrong, one of the senior psychiatrists in the department told me when I began my research. This reputation, he continued, was a draw for medical students wanting to learn psychiatry. Dr. Jackson, the director of resident education, confirmed that, when it comes to psychiatric training, medical students seek a "balance between training in psychotherapy and pharmacology."[1] But, he continued matter-of-factly, "most psychiatry residency programs say that they offer this balance." At Shorewood, these psychiatrists contended, "balance" was more than a promise.

An overview of the program supports their assertions. A brief description of the "didactic core curriculum" for psychiatry residents mentioned "balance" and its equivalents several times, including in a testimonial from a PGY-2 resident who declared, "I love how well our program achieves balance." Spread over four years, the curriculum consists of seminars covering a variety of topics ranging from psychiatric diagnosis to pharmacology to emergency psychiatry, consultation psychiatry, and psychotherapy. The commitment to epistemic equity is so important that, as the description makes clear, the same percentage of lecture time is devoted to neurobiology and diagnostic issues as is to psychodynamic and cognitive behavioral therapy. And, unlike less-resourced programs, Shorewood is well positioned to put such commitments into practice. It is part of one of the top university systems in the country and boasts faculty who do innovative research about the neurobiology of mental illnesses, while also maintaining connections to top psychology and social work departments. Shorewood has also preserved its historical ties to a local psychoanalytic institute, ties that have allowed it to revive its psychodynamic training for the residents three years before the Accreditation Council for Graduate Medical Education (ACGME) standards required it. Finally, the department has been home to an anxiety disorders clinic, bringing together, among others, experts in cognitive and behavioral treatments. As a whole, this indeed paints a "balanced" picture in today's psychiatric landscape.

Yet this programmatic and institutional "balance" should not be taken to mean that the residents training at Shorewood develop a symmetrical view of learning and doing pharmacological and talk therapeutic interventions. The timing and practical demands of biological and psychotherapeutic training indicate otherwise. In keeping with the broader field's priorities, much of the residents' education and clinical work is dedicated to mastering the neurobiology of mental illness and its pharmacological treatments. Moreover, even as they may come to Shorewood seeking a "balanced" program, their early and intensive immersion in hospital psychiatry cultivates a biological mindset. By the time their in-depth psychotherapy training begins in the third postgraduate year (PGY-3), psychiatry residents have already adopted a biomedical framework and professional identity.

Socialized to think of mental illness as a disease of the brain, and of themselves as psychopharmacologists, the residents begin psychotherapy training ill equipped to accept its radically distinct epistemic assumptions. Their path toward psychotherapeutic competence is further imperiled by the timing of its requirements: the residents begin therapy training just as they anticipate greater autonomy as medication prescribers during the middle stages of the program. Their roles are thus replete with epistemic and professional frictions. Skepticism is their inevitable corollary. These frictions and the early doubts that accompany them are heightened by the residents' job expectations. Just like the senior psychiatrists who train them, the residents are well aware that they are expected to write and manage medication prescriptions, even if they may wish to conduct psychotherapy. As essential as psychotherapy training is—for the program's accreditation, for the residents' performance on their board certification exams, and for patients' well-being—it is not viewed as equivalent to gaining pharmacological expertise. Even as he extolled Shorewood's "balanced approach," Dr. Armstrong reminded me that the program's psychotherapy offerings are not "designed to produce professional therapists." Instead, he explained, "we are socializing [the residents] to understand and respect professional therapists, but not necessarily to adopt that identity themselves." Psychotherapy remains at arm's length.

In this chapter, I begin the story of the residents' journeys from skepticism to competence with a discussion of the conditions that make skepticism an inevitable feature of their roles. I start with a brief overview of the program's history and a description of the residents' training over the four years of the adult psychiatry program. Their accumulated experiences converge on an essential idea—namely, that their primary epistemic and professional task is to manage mental illness through chemical means. By the time they start psychotherapy training as third years, the residents view it both as secondary to psychopharmacology and as the domain of psychologists and social workers. It is the job of Shorewood's psychotherapy instructors to convince them otherwise, even if only temporarily, and I introduce them and their goals next. I end the chapter with a discussion of the first and most enduring manifestation of the residents' contradictory demands: time. As they navigate the constraints of their training schedules, the residents are caught between their roles as medication prescribers and as psychotherapy trainees. The distinct expectations associated with these roles reflect the epistemic and professional friction the residents must navigate and create fertile conditions for skepticism.

Shorewood

Shorewood was established in the early 1900s as the "Department of Nervous and Mental Diseases," owing its existence to federal funding aimed at establishing mental hospitals around the country. In the 1920s, the psychiatry department formally came into being after splitting off from neurology. Under the leadership of an ambitious chair, it began a long period of expansion in both research and clinical arenas. Reflecting the national entrenchment of psychoanalysis in psychiatry after World War II (1939–45), Shorewood's hospital and clinic were dedicated to treating patients with the approach. Even the psychiatrists who conducted biological interventions such as insulin shock therapy or electroconvulsive therapy, or did research on what are now known as serious mental illnesses (e.g., schizophrenia), underwent psychoanalytic training at the local institute. Nevertheless, fissures in the system began to appear in the 1960s, as questions about how to implement the Community Mental Health Centers Act brought to light the department's emphasis on treating relatively less sick and more well-to-do patients.[2] The program was ill equipped to help those who suffered from chronic and highly debilitating conditions. It also lacked the space, time, and faculty to meet the demand for psychoanalytic services that it had helped create.

Akin to other psychiatry departments around the country, the 1960s and '70s were marked by crisis for the program and its residency. Even more than today, residents had to navigate their field's splintered identity. Divided between psychoanalysis, biological psychiatry, and social psychiatry, trainees had to find their own way while demonstrating some familiarity with each approach. Then, in the late 1970s, psychoanalysts were largely pushed out through a new requirement that all full-time university employees work solely for the university. As was common at the time, the majority of psychoanalytic psychiatrists also had private practices, and they chose those over the university.[3] The eventual rupture in Shorewood's relationships with the local psychoanalytic institute reflected the broader marginalization of psychoanalysis that culminated with the 1980 publication of the third edition of the *Diagnostic and Statistical Manual of Mental Disorders* (DSM-III) and the ouster of psychoanalysts from positions of power in universities around the US and at the American Psychiatric Association.

The appointment of a biologically oriented psychiatrist as department chair in the mid-1980s marked a definitive break with the psychoanalytic approach. It also brought coherence and a new direction to Shorewood and its residency program. Psychopharmacology quickly emerged as a solution to the problems that psychiatry was facing nationally and locally. Rising health care costs and the growing role of insurance companies in determining the kind and duration of treatments they would pay for transformed psychiatric practice and training. The key "lesson" the residents training at this time had to learn, a Shorewood psychiatrist wrote, was how to be most "efficient."[4] At the same time, psychiatry was seeking to become better aligned with the rest of medicine, receiving a boost during the 1990s "Decade of the Brain," as federal funding for research into the brain mechanisms underlying mental illnesses increased at Shorewood and elsewhere.[5] Concurrently, biopsychiatry became the dominant framework for educating residents across the country.

But, just as quickly as it had set in, this framework too began to shift. Early during my fieldwork, I spoke with Dr. Hoffman, a psychiatrist who had trained at Shorewood in the late 1990s. She explained to me that, in the decade before her arrival, the program did not offer residents any formal training in talk and behavioral interventions. They could pick it up if they worked with a psychodynamically inclined physician at the hospital, but otherwise their focus was on diagnosis, the management of hospitalized patients, and, most important, pharmacology. But, as psychiatric education came under scrutiny nationally, Shorewood too began to expand its training to include skills in patient care. This meant reintroducing psychodynamic training into the curriculum and turning it into a rotation that required the rekindling of relationships with local psychoanalysts.

Dr. Jackson, the residency training director at Shorewood when I was there in the early 2010s, had been at the helm of the training program since this earlier period of curricular change. Like most psychiatrists training during the last wave of psychoanalytic influence in psychiatry, he had learned psychodynamic psychotherapy while working with hospitalized patients during his residency in the early 1980s. He told me that he had been required to complete two thousand hours of psychodynamic case work and contrasted that with the two hundred hours required of the residents training in the first decade of the 2000s. Nevertheless, despite his extensive psychodynamic training, Dr. Jackson's professional career reflected the field's biological turn: his research and clinical work focused exclusively on the brain and pharmacology.

He joined the faculty at Shorewood in the 1990s, a time when the residency program had eliminated psychotherapy from its requirements. But, he told me, the residents trained then "were completely mechanistic in their approach, using checklists and other such methods." Because they did not learn psychotherapy, "they made no efforts to understand the patients and their environment." More troubling, as another psychiatrist involved in the residency told me, the trainees were completing program requirements, but some were failing their board examinations. Thus, Dr. Jackson explained, even though it had been "relatively easy to eliminate therapy training from the curriculum," he and his colleagues brought it back. They began with a psychodynamic class and ramped up offerings and requirements shortly before the ACGME was instituting such a change nationally. In its greater emphasis on psychotherapy, Shorewood was a harbinger of broader changes in psychiatric education.

Three reasons motivated the decision to bring back psychotherapy, Dr. Jackson explained. First, the program had access to sufficient faculty to offer such training. Psychologists and social workers could bring expertise in cognitive and behavioral approaches. A vibrant local psychoanalytic institute and community could offer support for psychodynamic training, and its members returned to teaching in the program with little fanfare. Accreditation standards constituted the second reason for formally re-introducing psychotherapy into the psychiatric curriculum. Shorewood anticipated and exceeded the ACGME standards. Commenting on the 2008 revision of the guidelines, Dr. Jackson explained that, whereas the rules were "really strict," programs have some leeway in how they implement them. The standards did not specify, he told me, "how much time needs to be spent on therapy training."[6] Moreover, the rules were "vague about what constitutes experience in therapy." For most psychiatry residencies, this is taken to mean "having some exposure to therapy, doing some consultations, but not much more." Yet at Shorewood, Dr. Jackson said, "we believe that some of these therapies are of enough value to our residents that we want them to train in [the approaches]."

This expressed belief in its value hinted at the third reason for Shorewood's greater commitment to psychotherapy. "The skills that the residents gain," Dr. Jackson stressed, "are very important." Although the residents would not get enough talk therapy training to become psychotherapists, "they are better doctors because of it." Dr. Jackson's comments in this respect reflected arguments made by other leaders in the field about why psychotherapy should not be expunged from the training of future psychiatrists.[7] They also fit with a broader reorientation in medicine toward training well-rounded doctors who are empathetic and can talk with their patients about their illness experiences.[8] In an ironic twist, psychiatry's connection to medicine no longer depended solely on its commitment to science and the brain. Psychotherapy could now play a role in that alignment, turning biopsychiatrists into "better doctors."

By the time I began my fieldwork at Shorewood, the program had been building its psychotherapeutic capacities for nearly ten years. It had reestablished connections with the local psychoanalytic institute by creating a robust psychodynamic training program, enlisting local analysts to serve as individual supervisors for the residents, paying the residents' fees should they wish to take classes at the institute, and making it possible for those who wanted to train as psychoanalysts to begin doing so before they completed the residency. I learned, to my surprise, that one or two residents per year still chose to do so. Moreover, rotations in cognitive behavioral therapy (CBT), dialectical behavioral therapy (DBT), and interpersonal psychotherapy (IPT) had been established shortly after the psychodynamic program got off the ground, with offerings in CBT expanding to accommodate a greater variety of disease-specific treatments. Finally, Shorewood's Child and Adolescent Psychiatry program is home to a vibrant research and clinical community that brings together biopsychiatric, psychodynamic, and cognitive behavioral experts. The residents could learn a broad range of therapies.

And this was precisely what I heard from both Dr. Jackson and the residents themselves. Dr. Jackson emphasized to me that, while the program meets accreditation standards, it is "very flexible and lets residents do training that is unique to their interests and needs." The residents, too, seemed to appreciate the approach. Leah, a resident I spoke with during her PGY-3, told me that she had chosen Shorewood because it afforded her "greater flexibility" to pursue topics she was interested in. This flexibility is most apparent in the final year of the residency (PGY-4), when the residents are provided "ample time" for "elective rotations," as Leah put it. Theoretically, this could mean that the residents could pursue more in-depth psychotherapy training. But, despite options and "balance," only a small minority did so. Why this was the case becomes clearer once we understand the structure of psychiatric training.

The (Bio)psychiatric Residency

The residency has become an almost necessary component of medical education for physicians practicing in the US.[9] Its length varies by specialty. The general psychiatry residency lasts three years following a one-year internship; residents can pursue additional education in a sub-specialty by completing one- or two-year fellowships in fields such as child and adolescent psychiatry, emergency psychiatry, or addiction psychiatry. During the residency, newly minted MDs learn how to interact with and take care of patients, develop the experience and confidence to practice independently, work with colleagues within and outside their specialty, deepen their medical knowledge, and acquire the moral and ethical toolkit of their profession. "It's in residency that you really sort of learn how to be a doctor," Lucas, a soon to be graduating fourth year (PGY-4), told me. And what kind of doctors the residents learn to be owes much to these early postgraduate years.

Akin to other medical fields, the transition from medical school to residency in psychiatry is marked by a yearlong internship. In the course of this transitional year (PGY-1), interns rotate through primary care settings (which may include internal medicine, pediatrics, or family medicine) as well as neurology and psychiatry.[10] Though no strangers to clinical work, medical students are relatively insulated from the kind of accountability that comes with the practice of medicine. The internship year plunges newly minted MDs into patient care and the responsibilities associated with it. It is during this time that they solidify their skills at taking patients' medical histories, collecting tissue and blood samples, writing admission notes, and devising treatment plans. All this happens in teams, under the close supervision of senior residents and *attendings*, experienced physicians who work in hospitals and oversee the work of trainees. Challenges abound. Helping dying or severely ill patients, all while doing the work of day-to-day medical care and navigating the demands of a new position in the professional hierarchy, proves grueling for many novice physicians. Nevertheless, by the end of this year, "the doctor feels like a doctor," as anthropologist T. M. Luhrmann put it.[11]

While interns have some exposure to psychiatry during the PGY-1, during the second postgraduate year (PGY-2)—the year that marks the formal start of the psychiatric residency—they work exclusively with psychiatric patients. At Shorewood, this meant rotating between the university-affiliated hospital and the hospital operated by the US Department of Veterans Affairs. Much of the residents' training at this time focuses on mastering psychiatric diagnoses and pharmacology. When Lucas, the PGY-4, told me about his work at the hospital, he did so by listing diagnoses: "There's a little bit of psychosis, sometimes you get some true mania, sometimes you get really severe Axis I depression, like really bad melancholia, you know, and they need to come in for an ECT [electroconvulsive therapy] or something like that." For Lucas, "inpatient psychiatry really is about becoming a specialist in a lot of personality disorders." He recalled that, on a day-to-day basis, he would "assess, and reassess, and reassess" patients at the hospital and, wittingly or not, "become an Axis II expert." As the resident's description implies, the hospital is a time for developing proficiency in diagnosis and the DSM.

Lucas's reference to Axis I and Axis II reflects his training prior to the 2013 publication of the DSM-5, which reshaped the classification of mental illnesses by eliminating the axial system.[12] Though this current version of the DSM lists diagnoses in order of clinical importance—with the most common, such as depression and anxiety, first—Lucas and his colleagues had learned to diagnose according to the previous version, the DSM-IV.[13] This earlier manual had them distinguish between Axis I diagnoses, which included the most prevalent mental health and substance use disorders, and Axis II, which encompassed personality disorders and mental retardation. Additionally, the residents had also learned to assess patients' other medical conditions (Axis III), their psychosocial and environmental problems (Axis IV), and overall functioning (Axis V). It was the first two categories that, by and large, preoccupied the budding psychiatrists, and for good reason: mood and personality disorders make up the core of psychiatry's jurisdiction.

But more than illustrating a historically contingent understanding of psychiatric diagnosis, Lucas's account of training at the hospital is also notable for being nearly devoid of patients. He talked of axes, diagnoses, symptoms, and treatments. With only days to spend with any given patient and up to twenty-five patients on the unit to oversee, the residents hardly had time to get to know the people cycling in and out of the psychiatric unit. Instead, they learned to think in categories. Patients' symptoms and their configuration into diagnoses dominated the trainees' imaginaries about what it meant to do psychiatry. Sandra, a recent Shorewood graduate, put it more starkly when she told me that she felt that the DSM was "stamped in [her] brain" from her years training in the hospital. It came up automatically when she spoke with patients about their troubles, even before she knew whether she would prescribe them medications.

Though he extolled Shorewood's psychotherapy offerings, Dr. Jackson was clear that "the first two years in the residency are about pharmacology." He explained, "About 90 percent [of the residents' time] is spent learning about it and doing it." For the junior residents, psychotropics could take on almost magical power. Sandra recalled that working on the psychiatry units as a PGY-2, she could see "what sounds outrageous come to life." She was fascinated by "psychotic patients [. . .] who were pretty delusional or grandiose, and *really* thought that they had special powers and could read my mind, and—and potentially fly if we let them try to jump." Yet even as such patients "might be [psychotic] for weeks," Sandra told me, "we could bring them down from it with a medication pretty quickly or easy [and] most of the time we could stop it." The experience of seeing patients respond to medications "was validating," Sandra explained. Working at the hospital convinced her, akin to her colleagues, that mental illness is biological and that psychiatry's chemical tools were the best ways to treat it.

The internship and the first year of residency were formative for the novice psychiatrists. The hospital circumscribed their attention and disciplined their thinking. It prepared them to be "efficient," as Dr. Hoffman put it. Patients arrived at the hospital severely sick and did not stay long. The residents' job was to return them to a state of relative independence and discharge them. They were training for a world where fifteen-minute "med management" appointments need to be spent ably translating patients' problems into the language and interventions of biological psychiatry. Significantly, the image of mental illness as a disease of the brain that can be diagnosed by assessing symptoms and treated with pharmaceuticals is a compelling professional worldview. Even Sandra, who had actually committed part of her practice to psychotherapy, would refer to the biological substrates of mental illness when discussing her reliance on psychotropic medications. Other psychiatrists who had chosen to practice psychotherapy after residency spoke in similar ways about their work. Such was the power of the hospital experience.

But the residents' deep commitment to biological psychiatry should not be taken for naivete. Lucas (PGY-4) reflected critically on his work at the hospital, asserting that "there are very, very few conditions in psychiatry that are amenable to quick fixes." He stressed that the inpatient unit was not a place of treatment but one where patients were "stabilized" with medications. "If somebody's having a true psychotic break, we can fix that in the short term. If somebody's really having a melancholic-type depression, you can see them in a couple weeks get dramatically better with ECT. If somebody's truly manic, you can see that come down in a couple weeks on the inpatient unit." Yet aside from these specific conditions, Lucas thought that patients' relative improvement in the hospital could be attributed to "nonspecific benefits," such as "being taken care of" and "the placebo effect of being given a medication."[14] The most commonly prescribed psychiatric medications, he told me, do not begin to show effects during the brief timeframe of a hospital stay.

Lucas was not alone in understanding the limitations of hospitalization and medications. During one therapy session I observed from behind a one-way mirror, Alayna (PGY-3) interviewed a young woman who had been hospitalized for an attempted suicide. Over her nine days at the hospital, the patient had received a new medication prescription. Two days after discharge, she quietly told Alayna that the new drugs had "made [her] feel better right away." Aaron, the PGY-3 I was sitting next to in the observation room, immediately turned to me and said, "Yeah, that doesn't happen. The meds don't work that fast. It's placebo effect and wishful thinking." As if on cue, Alayna asked her patient, "You already feel that?" This allowed the patient to discuss some of the more unpleasant effects of the new medication and admit that things had not been as good as she had initially described. The residents were prepared to recognize when the medications indeed worked and when it was merely patients' "wishful thinking." Patients, the residents learned, were "stabilized" in the hospital; drugs did not always work as patients—or the institutions charged with their care—"wished" they did.

The majority of the residents' time during the PGY-3 and PGY-4 was spent at Shorewood's outpatient clinic. The move from the hospital to the clinic marked a new stage in their training. One difference was that the number of patients they saw greatly expanded. Whereas in the hospital they had worked with a about two dozen patients, at the clinic they would "inherit" hundreds of patients from graduating residents. Moreover, their work shifted from crisis management to long-term care. The transition was not easy. Sandra recalled with a laugh that, as an early PGY-3, she "didn't like that patients [at the clinic] kind of roamed free [. . .] everywhere." Though not all patients were as "high acuity" as those whom she had treated at the hospital, it was hard to shake the caution she had developed there.

The new context did offer the residents some validation. At the clinic, they could work with patients for extended periods and, at times, see them get better. Lucas (PGY-4) told me that he had found that stage of the residency "much more satisfying" because it was at the clinic that "you can actually [. . .] modify the disease." No longer constrained to offer "quick fixes" where there were few, Lucas and his colleagues could focus on an illness's trajectory and its longer-term management. In turn, patients' improvement only affirmed the residents' belief in the biological vision of mental illness. After putting a younger patient on a common medication for attention deficit hyperactivity disorder (methylphenidate), Asha (PGY-4) remarked, "I'm actually surprised how much he's changed with just a little bit of Ritalin! I'm dazzled!" The hospital had not prepared the residents to see much progress from their patients. At the clinic, their pharmaceutical education could take on new meaning as they witnessed the positive effects of their chemical tools.

Practically, the residents' day-to-day work built on their inpatient years. Sandra described a typical appointment:

[Medication] appointments are often partially consumed with signing medication consent forms, and reviewing the side effects to medicines, and getting vitals, and those pieces of it, and lab work, and education on why I'm doing all of this. . . . [It's] primarily symptom guided. So, you know, if they had, you know, five symptoms of depression, are any of them better, or gone, or worse, or [are there] new ones? And kind of keeping track of which symptoms are changing.

Compared with hospital work, where the residents would see their patients every day, sometimes multiple times a day, pharmacology appointments were relatively infrequent, ranging from once a week in the early stage of treatment to once a month or once every six months during the "maintenance" stage. But, in content, pharmacology appointments required only a minor shift in professional practice. As Sandra made clear, the routine work of medication and symptom management had become deeply ingrained. The logic of symptoms, diagnoses, and prescriptions dictated the terms of interaction between patient and doctor, whether at the hospital or in the office.

And even as the residents also talked to patients about their lives and their experiences during prescription appointments, this was done with the relatively narrow purpose of understanding a medication's effects. Kyra, another recent Shorewood graduate, told me that she starts every pharmacology appointment by asking patients a question such as "How have things been going?" Patients' answers could help her learn about their quality of life and illness trajectories. Even so, should an open-ended approach result in a vague narrative, she would redirect the conversation. Kyra channeled her doctoring self as she demonstrated the gently assertive way she would guide such a patient: "Last time you were going to start BuSpar at 5 milligrams and go up to 10 milligrams. How did that go?" The task at hand was discerning the effects of medications on the patient's illness and overall "functioning," not how "things" in general have "been going."

Epistemically, one of the paradoxical processes that takes place as the residents advance in their training is that, just as their pharmacological competence solidifies, they became less bound by the DSM's diagnostic criteria.[15] Though a diagnosis may "influence what I might pick to prescribe first," Kyra told me, over time she would focus more on "getting to know the patient" and "seeing how they respond" to their medications. This focus is partly attributable to the nature of psychiatric diagnoses, as the same symptoms appear in different categories. It is also partly because of psychiatric medications themselves. Common SSRIs (selective serotonin reuptake inhibitors) are used to treat both depression and anxiety, even though these conditions have distinct designations in the DSM. Antipsychotics, typically used to treat psychosis, can be prescribed in combination with SSRIs in the treatment of severe depression or post-traumatic stress disorder, among other diagnoses.[16] Moreover, for reasons not yet understood, people respond in different ways to the same drugs, and psychiatrists try various medications until they find the prescription that works best for the particular patient. Symptoms rather than DSM diagnoses, and patients' own experiences taking the medications, guide psychiatrists, and the residents were becoming increasingly proficient at discerning such nuances.

It was in this context that they began their psychotherapy training as PGY-3s, entering the world of psychotherapy from a professional perspective sharpened by biological psychiatry. They felt unprepared for even the most basic tasks of talk and behavioral approaches. Andrew, a recent graduate, described as "scary" his first forays into psychotherapy. "You saw patients a certain way," he told me, referencing his hospital training, and "knew how to take a history, evaluate, diagnose, and prescribe a [medication] treatment." In psychotherapy, Andrew felt that he did not "have the tools" nor "the experience" to "really integrate what a patient [was] saying and where they're coming from." Unlike pharmacological work, which had become ingrained, doing psychotherapy was like being "on a high wire without a net." Psychotherapy training thrust the residents into a professional world they were ill equipped to navigate. Friction and skepticism were the inevitable effects of their new positions.

Though skeptical of psychotherapy and of the necessity of training in it, the residents knew that pharmacology did not have all the answers. Indeed, their biological training had prepared them to understand the hurdles they faced as practitioners in an uncertain field. Whether they came to see the DSM as only an imperfect device for capturing patients' suffering, or medications as imprecise tools for healing it, their belief in biological psychiatry's power was not absolute. Though they could point to the successes they experienced with pharmaceutical treatments, the residents also encountered plenty of frustrations. Time and again, they would discuss their patients' "breakthrough" symptoms on various SSRIs, the shortcomings of antipsychotics for treating delusions, or the outright failure of medications—even when administered together—to lessen patients' misery. Indeed, becoming an expert in this field was thus partly about recognizing its limitations. The residents were adept at doing so. They were able to display their proficiency in pharmacology not only through confident pronouncements about which drug might help a particular patient get better but also through knowing explanations of a drug's limitations and disadvantages. Being dogmatic about a particular approach was difficult given the residents' professional stage and the broader unsettledness of psychiatric knowledge.

Psychotherapy could help when chemical interventions proved of limited value. But the residents had few opportunities to learn this different way of doctoring early in the program. At the hospital, the best they could do was offer patients "supportive therapy," a combination of empathy and validation, in addition to a prescription. At times, they could participate in group therapy meetings. Lucas recalled that one of the problems he encountered during his time caring for hospitalized patients was that "oftentimes . . . you feel like a person really needs therapy, but our system isn't necessarily working into that." Even as later in the second postgraduate year the residents could begin psychodynamic treatments with one or two patients, there were few structural incentives or opportunities to do so. Lucas made clear that "certainly, you as the doctor, are not [at the hospital] to deliver [psychotherapy]." Instead, "social workers do that and the [therapy] group leaders do that." The residents quickly understood the constraints imposed on their positions by the professional and economic arrangements in their field.

Constraints also remained at the clinic, where the residents formally began training in psychotherapy. "There's no way in the system," Zoli (PGY-4) told me, "for people to get referred to me just for therapy." Even while working on an outpatient basis, "as an MD," Zoli could not do "split therapy," as he described it. He and his colleagues could treat patients with psychotherapy only if they also managed their pharmacological needs. The arrangement challenged the residents to navigate, sometimes with patients in real time, their contradictory positions.[17] Whereas more experienced psychiatrists can choose to treat their patients either pharmacologically or therapeutically, trainees did not always have the option to "separate" the two, as Zoli put it. They could be solely medication prescribers, but they could not be solely psychotherapists.[18]

Despite these constraints, psychotherapy took enough of the residents' time to constitute a significant aspect of their education. They began learning the basics of psychodynamic psychotherapy during the second postgraduate year, when they were also encouraged to start treating a patient in this approach. Some did so toward the end of their time at the hospital; most waited until the beginning of their time at the clinic as PGY-3s. Starting in the third postgraduate year, the residents were expected to treat two or three patients psychodynamically, meet weekly with the psychoanalysts who served as their individual supervisors, and also attend the weekly discussions of the psychodynamic core class. Additionally, they could also sign up for six-month rotations in CBT for anxiety or CBT for depression, DBT, IPT, or couples and marital therapy, each led by a psychologist or clinical social worker. Akin to the psychodynamic core class, meetings in these rotations took place once a week, but they lasted two hours instead of one. Unlike the psychodynamic rotation, these were open to psychology and social work trainees who were completing internships or fellowships at the clinic or working in some capacity with the instructor. In their third and fourth postgraduate years (PGY-3 and PGY-4), the residents spent several hours a week seeing such patients in psychotherapy, writing up therapy notes, meeting with psychotherapy supervisors, and attending didactic lectures on various approaches.

Though psychotherapy was a key source of stress for the residents during PGY-3, it became less so during their final year in the psychiatry program. On the one hand, the PGY-4 offered them more freedom to pursue their interests and potentially spend less time in psychotherapy. At Shorewood, this could mean learning about forensic psychiatry or consultation and liaison psychiatry, conducting research, or working at a local shelter for the unhoused. Some of the residents had already started their training in child and adolescent psychiatry as PGY-3s, while others prepared for fellowships in subspecialties such as addiction psychiatry, geriatric psychiatry, forensic psychiatry, sleep medicine, or pain medicine. On the other hand, and more essential to the story this book tells, as PGY-4s, the residents had developed some competence in talk and behavioral interventions and felt less encumbered by epistemic or professional friction. They could move between the worlds of biology and psychotherapy with greater freedom and ease.

Psychotherapy Instructors and Their Approaches

Much of the work of introducing residents to psychotherapy and convincing them of its value fell on their instructors in therapeutic rotations. Jeremy, a psychologist who had started the CBT training program at Shorewood and garnered multiple teaching awards along the way, led the CBT for anxiety rotation. To learn psychotherapies for depression, the residents could either pair up with Robert, a psychologist who ran the CBT for depression mentorship, or Holly, a psychologist and expert in IPT. The residents learned DBT, an approach designed for patients with longstanding mood instability and those diagnosed with borderline personality disorder, from Nora, an experienced social worker and an excellent therapist who, many thought, could get patients better when nobody else could. Finally, on the child and adolescent side, I spent time with Miriam's

CBT group, which met for three hours every week to discuss cases and conduct sessions in rooms equipped with one-way mirrors. Miriam is an experienced social worker with expertise in treating anxiety disorders in children.

These instructors, akin to Terry and Patricia, their counterparts in the psychodynamic rotation, had to shift the residents' thinking about what ailed their patients and how they could be best helped. Jeremy stressed that, in CBT, the residents would learn how to "find ways to get people to confront what they are afraid of," whether through behavioral interventions or thought exercises. "Our job in cognitive therapy," he later explained, "is to help [patients] think about [their problems] in a more reasonable way." At the hospital, residents tended to focus on the "reasonableness" of their patients' thinking only as a symptom, typically of psychosis. In CBT, they would have to travel to the more confounding domain of fostering "reasonableness" through cognitive and behavioral exercises.

Nevertheless, compared with their psychodynamic colleagues, instructors in these approaches faced an easier mandate. For one, some of these interventions shared affinities with biopsychiatry that lessened the epistemic friction the residents confronted. And, while these instructors did encourage their trainees, even strongly, to find patients with whom they would conduct the particular approach, they infrequently made it an open point of contention, thus minimizing opportunities for professional friction. Instead, they focused on teaching residents how to integrate the skills they were learning into medication management appointments. Moreover, they wanted to equip the psychiatrists with the epistemic generosity needed to work in multidisciplinary teams that included several types of mental health care providers. Nora explained to the residents that her broader goal was to prepare them to let go of some of their authority as "prescribers" and learn to occupy a more "supportive role" for the therapists who actually conducted DBT, typically psychologists and social workers. Even with DBT "concepts" and "strategies" in their tool kit, the residents would not become therapists. The division of labor would remain undisturbed.

Matters were more complicated in psychodynamic training. The task of helping the residents work through their skepticism and develop a modicum of competence in the approach fell on two trained psychoanalysts, Terry, a psychiatrist, and Patricia, a psychologist. In contrast to learning CBT and related interventions, the residents' training in psychodynamic psychotherapy started during the second postgraduate year. While they were still working at the hospital, the residents would gather in a conference room over an "allotted" eight meetings during the course of the year to learn the basics of the approach from the two psychoanalysts. When I spoke with Terry and Patricia about their goals, they converged on wanting the residents to develop a new way of understanding their patients, "as more than just chemicals," in Terry's words. They hoped that the residents would come to "see the patient as a person," Patricia explained, and recognize how their own identities and emotions shape what they "see."

I tagged along with Terry on his first meeting with a group of PGY-2s. Over coffee and pastries, Terry used a mixture of humor, cultural references, didactics, and clinical material to ease the residents into the world of psychodynamic psychotherapy. The approach, Terry noted at the start of the discussion, is "the one opportunity [. . .] that we all have to sit back and sort of appreciate the patients." In contrast to the harried rhythms of hospital work, psychodynamic psychotherapy would give the residents time to listen to and "appreciate" their patients. Yet what this might mean remained obscure for the PGY-2s, worried as they were about their suicidal or psychotic patients on the wards. These residents did not yet have the kind of flexible epistemic imaginaries that their more advanced colleagues had developed to "appreciate" their patients beyond their presenting problems, symptoms, and medication regimens.

Aware of the contrasting epistemic and professional worlds the residents were inhabiting, Terry began to bridge the gap during the meeting. He spent the better part of an hour giving a broad overview of psychoanalysis, covering the basics of psychoanalytic theory—the theory of mind, theories of development—all the while making references to neuroscientific research. His approach seemed perfectly calibrated to his audience: he did not turn Freud into a visionary nor was he uncritical of psychoanalytic theories themselves, thus signaling his own rejection of the dogmatic stance sometimes associated with psychoanalysis. But he did not renounce the core tenets of psychoanalysis either. After a few minutes explaining Freud's conception of drives, Terry asked, "And the drives and instincts in the biz are referred to as what?" Several residents murmured "id" in response. "Those are the drives that seek satisfaction, such as hunger, comfort, sex, love, aggression, competition," Terry continued. Then he sought to bridge psychoanalysis with the residents' brain-based understanding of the mind: "Think of it neuroscientifically; where would those [drives] fit in, physiologically? So we call it the id from a psychological standpoint. What would we call it from a neurophysiologic standpoint? Where would that stuff hang out?" One of the residents chimed in, "In the limbic system." The connection was made. Psychoanalysis, at least in Terry's telling, was not that far from the neurobiological science the residents were learning. For the residents, such connections helped legitimize psychodynamic psychotherapy even as they did not fully erase the epistemic and practical gap between it and their hospital work.

Terry and Patricia set up structures to ease the residents' transition to the more intensive part of their psychodynamic training in the third postgraduate year: they paired them with psychoanalysts who served as their supervisors, helped them find patients they could work with psychodynamically, and ran the weekly discussion group. They guided them through psychoanalytic theory and offered them practical advice about how to talk to patients, how to think about their problems, and how to manage the dilemmas of being a doctor and a person at the same time. They encouraged the residents to take on more psychodynamic patients and work more intensively with them.

But the residents were not Terry's and Patricia's only interlocutors when it came to psychodynamic training. The psychoanalysts, akin to instructors in other therapeutic approaches, were also engaged in a dialogue about the necessity and extent of such training with departmental leadership. And while at the time CBT, DBT, and IPT were on more secure footing, the psychodynamic program was more closely scrutinized because it demanded more of the residents' time than any other talk and behavioral approach. In this context, the residents' competence in psychodynamic psychotherapy could be granted outsized importance. At the time, the residents' knowledge was formally assessed with the aid of the Psychodynamic Psychotherapy Competency Test.[19] Developed by a group of Columbia University psychiatrists, the test was intended to evaluate psychiatry residents' facility with psychodynamic concepts and their clinical applications and included vignettes that needed to be parsed out in multiple-choice questions. Terry viewed the test as more than a way of judging the residents' knowledge. It was also, he told me, a tool for evaluating the quality of the psychodynamic training program. Together with Patricia, he would discuss the results with Dr. Jackson, the residency director, and decide on programmatic changes deemed necessary for improving the residents' skills.

I observed Terry and Patricia do a practice session with the trainees, and I was struck by what a poor indicator of practical psychodynamic competence the test was. The residents' answers betrayed their limited knowledge: they could not always articulate the meaning of some of the concepts and infrequently chose the correct options among those offered. Reflecting on what had gone wrong, Terry was dismayed that the residents didn't "trust their own experiences," wanting instead "the books and the theories." In other words, the novices wanted to learn definitions and conceptual rules, whereas Terry had hoped that they would draw on the "practical wisdom" they would have begun developing while treating their patients psychodynamically. For their part, the residents were unsure about how they could connect their clinical experience with knowledge of psychoanalytic concepts. Terry later told me that they "didn't do so well" on the actual test. When the results came back lower than they had expected, Terry and Patricia worked with Dr. Jackson to institute a more structured didactic curriculum in the first two years of the residency.

Though they used the test to improve the residents' training, Terry and Patricia worried about what the results indicated about the trainees' own priorities. During a conversation we had shortly after the end of my field-work, Terry wondered whether the residents' poor performance could be partly explained by "the possibility that they think that none of this stuff is worthwhile." The junior psychiatrists' ambivalence toward psychotherapy generally, and psychodynamic psychotherapy in particular, was indisput-able. But, whether or not they thought psychotherapy was worthwhile, their growing competence also became evident over time. Terry and Pa-tricia, too, noticed a change in how the more advanced residents talked about their patients, displaying "introspection" and understanding "their role in eliciting the patient's reactions," in Terry's words. Competence was not simply the domain of test taking. Rather, as I will show in chapter 7, it is performed in case discussions and case presentations.

In sum, compared to other programs, Shorewood offered its residents multiple opportunities to learn psychotherapy. The core curriculum ex-posed them to a variety of mental health interventions, with time set aside for talk and behavioral approaches. Nevertheless, there was agreement among the program's leaders, the psychotherapy instructors, and the res-idents themselves that this training was not intended to turn them into psychotherapists. Rather, it was to equip them with the epistemic imagi-naries and tools that would allow them to recognize when a patient needed something other than medications and either implement the alternative treatment or, more commonly, find a therapist who would. But despite this seemingly straightforward setup, challenges remained.

The Constraints of Time and the Residents' Early Encounters with Friction

Time is a precious and limited resource for medical trainees, one that requires intensive and persistent management.[20] It is also a symbol of the friction that novices and professionals alike must navigate. As the resi-dents started in their roles as psychotherapy novices, they faced new and incompatible demands that frequently coalesced around their schedules. The contradictions embedded in their positions were particularly appar-ent when they needed to set aside their psychiatric commitments and turn to learning psychotherapy instead. At the hospital, the PGY-2s strug-gled to get away from their clinical duties to attend didactic lectures in psychodynamic psychotherapy, even as, in principle, time was set aside for these lectures. Though the residents' schedules were clearly delineated, actually implementing them and doing so productively remained a challenge.

But attending such lectures alone would not guarantee a smooth transition between the world of the hospital and that of psychotherapy. Sanjay (PGY-3) explained that at the hospital "my thoughts are at the level of, 'does this person have delirium because they have an infection?'" Patients' relational patterns, much less their unconscious conflicts, were far from the residents' "thoughts." The "boundary" of the residents' "knowledge," as Sanjay described it, was such that the epistemic gulf between thinking medically and thinking psychodynamically only heightened the feeling of being short on time. Instead of psychoanalytic theory, the residents wanted practical tips: How do you talk to a patient when you first meet them? Can you take notes? How do you ask about painful or taboo experiences? The residents wanted to know how they could help their patients when drugs were off the table.

Managing time became more complicated during the third postgraduate year. The year encapsulated the tension between the program's image as "balanced" and "flexible" and the reality of training in a field configured around pharmacology. The residents were required to attend the psychodynamic rotation and could choose among the other approaches, though, as Leah (PGY-3) told me, "you are not guaranteed to get what you want," as some of the rotations were more popular than others, and not all the residents got the placement they hoped for. The residents had "protected time"—time scheduled in advance—for the weekly meetings of the psychodynamic core class and other psychotherapy rotations. But they also faced intense pressures to set time aside for "return visits," as medication appointments were known, at the clinic. Moreover, they did not have protected time to read assigned materials or do psychotherapy "homework." Nor did they have one-hour blocks set aside for scheduling psychotherapy sessions with patients. Between the generous thirty minutes they could use for medication management appointments and the one- or two-hour blocks scheduled for various didactic activities and "clinics," the residents had difficulties finding the one-hour intervals necessary for psychotherapy.[21]

Their instructors were aware of such conundrums. During the first meeting of IPT, Holly repeatedly stressed the importance of working with a patient to learn the approach. "One of the greatest barriers for the residents," Holly explained to the group, was finding "one hour in their schedules to fit a patient." Indeed, by the end of their six months in the rotation, none of the residents who were there had conducted an IPT treatment—a lack of experience that constituted a major impediment to achieving competence in the approach. Few did so in the cognitive and behavioral rotations. But, because both CBT and DBT revolved principally around specific techniques and tools, the residents focused on integrating them into their medication management sessions. For their part, psychotherapy instructors in these orientations did not object to this solution, even encouraging the residents to adopt it when seeing patients exclusively for therapy was not possible.

Psychodynamic training required a greater temporal commitment. In addition to participating in the psychodynamic group's weekly meetings, the residents were required to treat multiple patients and meet with their psychoanalytic supervisors. Temporal and normative challenges regularly cropped up, particularly around how many patients the residents ought to see and how frequently they should meet with them. The ideal, from Terry's and Patricia's perspective, was treating three patients, including one male and one female, and doing so with a frequency of three sessions a week. Not quite psychoanalysis, the arrangement would have required the residents to set aside nine hours in their weekly schedules for psychodynamic treatment alone, in addition to the hour dedicated to the psychodynamic group and the one for supervision. This time commitment, many of the residents thought, was unworkable.

I heard about the residents' temporal troubles early in my fieldwork. Ryder (PGY-3) shared a conundrum: he had two psychodynamic patients and was contemplating meeting with each twice a week.

> The problem I'm having with that is, if I book them each, that's gonna cut down my available hours for other [medication management] people. So my [psychoanalytic] supervisor is pretty adamant, you have to see them twice a week! The patients are kind of on the fence about it because of scheduling and vacations coming up over the summer, and I guess I'm a little uncomfortable because I would probably have to extend my hours to see other people. So, what do you . . . ? . . . [My supervisor] was even telling me to try to do three times a week and that's really impossible for me to fit that in!

Ryder faced a common problem: at the clinic he was expected to have a certain number of hours available for psychopharmacology patients. Draymond, a PGY-3 at the time, pointed out that the financial incentives of the "system" made it such that they were "encouraged to get . . . nonpsychotherapy, just general patients for half-hour [med management] visits." Taking on additional patients for psychodynamic psychotherapy and increasing session frequency from once to twice or even three times a week put the residents in an "impossible" position. Ryder would have "to extend [his] hours" to fit both his pharmacology and his psychotherapy patients into his schedule.[22]

Both PGY-3s and PGY-4s complained frequently about these temporal pressures. Their psychiatric duties at Shorewood were seemingly immutable. Their medication management schedules, filled months in advance, were relatively inflexible. But they had to make time for psychodynamic psychotherapy patients, not to mention patients for the other therapy approaches they learned. Their instructors advised or, as was the case in psychodynamic training, required it, and their psychoanalytic supervisors applied similar pressure in their weekly meetings. The residents made compromises, but most would simply do less therapy than what their instructors and supervisors expected. Terry stressed that "the experience of working with a patient over a year, more than once a week, is critical." A small minority of residents conducted treatments with one patient in the highly recommended format of three times a week and testified to the usefulness of the experience. Most did not.

Without enough time to meet the demands of psychotherapy training, the residents found shortcuts. Most treated two psychodynamic patients in once-weekly meetings. They agreed with Andrea's (PGY-3) implicit stance: "I think that the three [psychodynamic] patient expectation is . . ." She did not need to finish her sentence. It was clear that she thought that the requirement to take on three patients whom she should see multiple times a week in psychodynamic psychotherapy was untenable. And while Terry and Patricia attributed the residents' reluctance to do more psychodynamic psychotherapy to what they "valued" in their education, Vinit, a PGY-4, described it as structural: "If [meeting with patients multiple times a week] is such a vital part of learning this therapy, it would be nice to have that part [of our training time] protected." Psychotherapy instructors' expectations ran counter to Shorewood's and the broader field's priorities. The residents were caught in the middle and had to devise ways to manage the friction embedded in their roles.

Conclusion

At Shorewood, the residents entered a program committed to exposing them to a range of psychotherapeutic approaches.[23] They could learn psychodynamic psychotherapy, work closely with local psychoanalysts, and even begin psychoanalytic training if they wished. They could also learn CBT, DBT, IPT, and couples and marital counseling. All the while, they became increasingly competent in biological psychiatry, learning to diagnose and prescribe. Nevertheless, despite the program's image as "balanced" and "flexible," the residents' time and attention were not equally distributed among approaches. Though a standout for its therapeutic offerings, Shorewood, akin to the broader field of psychiatry, remains committed to the biological understanding and treatment of mental illness.

This commitment is evident in the organization of the residents' time. Their first two years after medical school (PGY-1 and PGY-2) are dedicated to hospital work. Caring for severely ill patients whose treatment centers on medications socializes the residents to think of mental illness as a disease of the brain. This period is thus marked by a further entrenchment of the biomedical perspective that had become already established in medical school. They come to psychotherapy at a point in their training when they feel they have acquired a modicum of expertise in psychiatric pharmacology. It is also a time when they anticipate greater autonomy, as the residents shift from working on the inpatient units to having private offices at the clinic where they meet with patients away from the gaze of senior physicians. In this context, psychotherapy training poses the residents both epistemic and professional challenges. They need to learn distinct ways to doctor and accommodate to new role constraints. The latter find their earliest expression in the residents' struggles for time. Between medication appointments scheduled far in advance and clinical rotations that take up entire days, the psychiatrists have few opportunities to adapt to the temporal demands of conducting therapy. Caught between the worlds of biopsychiatry and psychotherapy, most residents chose the path of least resistance: taking on fewer therapy patients but fulfilling their program-mandated duties.

The residents' solution to the structural ambivalence stemming from their roles as psychiatrists training in psychotherapy reflects their profession's priorities as much as their own. On the one hand, their temporal constraints symbolize psychiatry's priorities, which currently center on preparing professionals who·can put into practice the dominant vision of mental illness as a disease of the brain. Psychotherapy instructors' own limited ability to enforce particular expectations around training and the time residents should dedicate to it further attest to talk and behavioral interventions' lower standing in the psychiatric profession. On the other hand, the residents' struggles to craft a path for themselves in the face of pressures from the program and from their psychotherapy instructors can be viewed as constitutive of the broader project of developing autonomous professional identities. They could not outright ignore their psychotherapy training, just as they could not evade their duties at the clinic. Nevertheless, these contradictory roles functioned within a biopsychiatric ecosystem that matched the residents' own expectations for their future career paths as pharmacologists, giving them a modicum of independence vis-à-vis psychotherapy training.

Not fully independent, nor fully subordinate, the residents were what I came to think of as professional novices. They had had enough training to be trusted with performing their professional duties autonomously. Even so, as they began psychotherapy training, they were thrust in the position of neophytes in need of instruction and supervision. Dilemmas of time were one of the earliest and most persistent manifestations of their contradictory roles. Sociologists have noted that the distribution and organization of time is socially patterned such that social actors in higher-status positions have greater control over their own and others' time than those in lower-status positions.[24] From this perspective, the residents' temporal conundrums can be viewed as their attempts at shedding the "novice" label and asserting the more preferable status of "professional." Their struggles underscored the friction they had to navigate.

Despite these structural problems, the residents understood the clinical utility of learning psychotherapy. Their pharmacological expertise was not simply about knowing when and how to prescribe medications. It was also about understanding the limits of biological interventions, limits that became evident when patients did not get better with pharmaceutical regimens alone. The boundary zone between biological psychiatry and psychotherapy was thus not only a space of friction but also one of possibility. Yet taking advantage of the epistemic opportunities opened up by therapeutic approaches required the residents to set aside some of their existing assumptions and practices and I turn to the challenges of doing so next.

3 * Doctoring Unmoored

"At first, when I got my [psychotherapy] patient, I had no idea how the mechanics of this work," Sanjay (PGY-3) admitted during a discussion in the psychodynamic rotation. Turner (PGY-3), too, revealed feeling "a little bit lost" when he began to work psychodynamically. The approach, he explained, "is pretty dramatically different" from what he was used to doing at the hospital. "The model" there, Turner continued, was that "you come in with pieces of information" about the patient, "make a decision" about their diagnosis and course of medication, "and then once you make a decision, you leave. You might spend thirty minutes with this person who needs more time, [but] you don't even have any concept about how to deal with an outpatient where you're trying to use the time for therapy." The residents knew how to assess "the treatment, the medication issues, the symptoms." In psychotherapy, they would have to set aside much of what they had come to take for granted about what it means to doctor.

Chapter 2 showed how the organization of psychiatric training fostered the epistemic and professional friction the residents experienced as they began to learn psychotherapy. Sanjay, Turner, and their colleagues had spent the previous two years mastering biomedical approaches to mental illness in the hospital. In their third postgraduate year (PGY-3), they continued to deepen that knowledge partly by working at the outpatient clinic as psychopharmacologists. But just as they became increasingly anchored in biological psychiatry, the residents started training in psychotherapy, needing to make space for new epistemic practices and professional roles. This laid the groundwork for unmooring their doctoring approach and inciting their skepticism.

This chapter begins to elucidate the residents' dilemmas by focusing on two problems that encapsulated the frictions they faced. Epistemically, the psychiatrists find that their basic assumptions about mental illness have little traction in psychotherapy, and the first part of the chapter shows them struggling with this growing realization. On the one hand, they discover that their biomedical knowledge of diagnosis and symptoms is considered either insufficient (in cognitive behavioral therapy [CBT]) or outright misguided (in psychodynamic therapy). On the other hand, the residents come to see that psychotherapeutic approaches privilege patients' accounts of their illnesses in ways that contradict their biopsychiatric training. With little use for their existing tools, and a shrinking sense of epistemic authority, the residents begin to voice their skepticism as they confront the friction between what they know and what they are learning.

Professionally, the residents find themselves compelled to occupy the position of psychotherapy novices, even as they move toward greater autonomy in their roles as psychopharmacologists at the clinic. Their training in psychotherapy takes place principally through conversations with instructors and supervisors. Though important conduits of new knowledge, these relationships also encapsulate the residents' structurally ambivalent roles. In the latter part of the chapter, I describe their conundrums as professional novices and show them chafing at their prolonged subordination. Even as they depend on psychotherapy instructors and supervisors for guidance, the residents also seek to assert their growing authority and autonomy. Here too, skepticism is the inevitable result of role contradictions. Its expression through displays of doubt helps the residents assert a modicum of control over their positions.

Epistemic Friction

Early in their training, the residents had learned to rely on the *Diagnostic and Statistical Manual of Mental Disorders* (known familiarly as the DSM) and its checklists to make sense of their patients' problems. As they began psychotherapy training, this knowledge proved of little utility. In this part of the chapter, I show them confronting the limitations of their diagnostic tools in the world of psychotherapy. First, the residents are repeatedly told that the DSM does little to reveal patients' thought and behavioral problems or their relational and unconscious conflicts. Second, I show the residents becoming increasingly troubled by their dependence on patients for access to their inner lives, their principal object of knowledge in psychotherapy. In this context, the residents struggle to maintain their earlier assurance and perceive their epistemic authority diminish. This, in turn, activates their skepticism, and they turn to expressions of doubt to anchor their sense of worth.

UNSETTLING DIAGNOSTIC THINKING

Diagnosis is one of the key skills residents acquire during psychiatric training. During medical school and the early years of residency they learn the criteria associated with DSM categories and develop aptitudes for identifying and classifying symptoms. In psychotherapy, the residents find that the DSM is of limited utility.[1] While they had already begun to think more flexibly about diagnosis in pharmacology, patients' symptoms remained an important focus. But, the residents would learn, symptoms, too, were of little psychotherapeutic use. No matter how practical they were—for patients, for insurers, for hospital administrators, and for the residents themselves—DSM diagnoses and their accompanying symptoms could obscure as much as they revealed. Knowing that someone suffered from major depressive disorder (DSM-5 codes 296.36–296.24) did not illuminate the patient's thoughts, feelings, and behaviors to a CBT practitioner, nor did it tell a psychodynamic psychotherapist why the patient suffered. In talk and behavioral approaches, the residents would have to recalibrate their expectations about how they can make sense of their patients' problems.

DSM Diagnoses as Necessary but Insufficient in CBT

Cognitive behavioral therapy placed the residents on more recognizable terrain. Just as in biopsychiatry, they found diagnosis to be an organizing principle of treatment in CBT. The very configuration of training in this approach made clear that diagnosis mattered: during the time of my observations, CBT groups were split by the two most common disease clusters in adults: depression and anxiety. And although the residents frequently found that their patients suffered from both depression and anxiety—thus challenging the neat separation between diagnoses and their treatments—symptoms remained an important means for determining a course of treatment. Just as in their pharmacological work, in CBT the residents continued to rely on diagnostic instruments to assess patients' symptoms; some of the most commonly used include the Beck inventories for depression or anxiety, the Hamilton scales for depression or anxiety, variations on the Patient Health Questionnaire, or the Generalized Anxiety Disorders questionnaire. Such forms were the material manifestations of overlaps between biopsychiatric and cognitive behavioral approaches when it came to understanding patients' suffering.

The import of diagnosis became especially clear during a treatment I observed as part of a CBT rotation focused on children and adolescents. Miriam, the clinical social worker who ran the rotation, led a group of trainees that included two psychiatry residents completing their fellowships in child psychiatry, seven social work interns, and two midcareer social workers seeking additional certification. Over the course of six months, I joined them as they watched and discussed treatments conducted by some of the group's members with younger patients. Sessions took place in a sparsely furnished room outfitted with a large one-way mirror. Along with Miriam and some of the trainees, I would sit in the dark, crammed observation room, watching the sessions unfolding under the bright fluorescent lights on the other side of the glass. The silence in the observation room was frequently interrupted by one or another member of the group commenting on a patient's or therapist's demeanor or reacting to the action unfolding before them. At times, Miriam would offer hushed commentary on the session or send short messages via a pager to the therapist in action, suggesting questions or comments they could ask the patient.

One such treatment involved Sam, a young man nearing eighteen who, as was typical in this age group, had come to the clinic at the urging of his family. Sonora (PGY-4), the resident who would be his therapist, had already completed one year of internship and two years in an adult residency program; she was now in her first year of the fellowship in child and adolescent psychiatry. Sam seemed shy and kept mostly quiet during their first session. His parents did much of the talking: earlier in the year, Sam had had trouble doing his schoolwork because of what they called his "perfectionism." He had been proud of his handwriting in the past, but it had become an obsession: Sam would spend hours perfecting the lines and curves on the page, falling further behind in his classes. His problem, diagnosed by his family and a previous therapist, was obsessive-compulsive disorder (OCD).[2]

The members of the training group looked forward to working on OCD and implementing its corresponding exposure and response prevention (ERP) treatment: it was one of Miriam's areas of expertise and could lend itself to swift success. Yet when Sonora administered the OCD diagnostic inventory during her next session alone with Sam, doubts emerged. Sam was not as concerned about his handwriting as it initially seemed. It was summer, and he was doing less of it than when school was in session. He also did not seem to engage in the "safety" behaviors typical of the OCD diagnosis, nor did he have the catastrophic fears that are known to motivate those who suffer from the illness. Additionally, Sam was so quiet and his comments so terse that it was hard to believe he was giving a complete account of his problems. After the diagnostic sessions, Miriam explained to Sonora and the rest of the group that "it's not unusual for kids or people with OCD to minimize their symptoms," partly because they know "that we're gonna ask [them] to do something unpleasant."

By the end of their five months together, Sonora would be unable to pin down Sam's diagnosis or the specific thoughts that she could target with CBT tools. Treatment was a guessing game littered with doubts about what Sam actually suffered from, why he came to therapy, and what, if anything, he was getting out of it. The group came to think that Sam was actually worried about his social life during the new academic year and, especially, about his sexual orientation. Having grown up in a strictly religious household, these concerns fueled his symptoms. Yet in a treatment approach where interventions are tightly linked to symptoms and diagnoses, Sonora could hardly help Sam get better with CBT techniques. For his part, Sam did eventually seem to benefit from their meetings, but not quite in the ways that Sonora and the CBT team had anticipated. Sonora's steadiness, openness, and acceptance seemed to help him more than any of the exposure exercises they had devised but Sam never completed.

Sonora's conundrums with Sam are emblematic of the importance that CBT practitioners attach to understanding patients' suffering through the lens of symptoms and diagnoses. However, it quickly became evident during discussions I observed in CBT rotations that diagnosis was only the first step toward treatment. Indeed, the residents had to move beyond a focus on classification and learn to identify patients' particular patterns of thinking, feeling, and acting. For example, OCD was one of the most commonly discussed illnesses in the rotation on CBT for anxiety in adults. But, of four patients diagnosed with OCD whose treatments came up for discussion in close succession, one had problems with recurring sexual and violent thoughts, another was concerned about accidentally bumping into people and gravely injuring them, and the remaining two were tormented by personal "imperfections" and turned to prayer to mitigate them. Despite their similarities, however, the latter two had disparate reasons for resorting to prayer: one was worried about her sexual behaviors while the other was focused on caring for his siblings.

These differences were consequential for treatment, and the residents had to attend to the unique constellations of thoughts and behaviors that motivated each patient's symptoms to craft appropriate interventions. All the patients who had been diagnosed with OCD received the same ERP treatment that had them engage in the activities that provoked their fears (exposure) but forgo their fear management strategies (response prevention). Yet each treatment looked different depending on patients' thoughts and behaviors. For the patient with recurring sexual and violent thoughts, treatment began with listening to recordings of herself voicing the repetitive thoughts that terrified her, continued with doing so while holding sharp objects, followed by holding sharp objects and looking at sexually suggestive images, and so on. The patient who was worried about accidentally injuring those around him received treatment that included walking in tight spaces and around corners in the presence of others. The two praying patients had to engage in "minor imperfections," as Jeremy, the psychologist who ran the CBT for anxiety rotation, put it, and such "imperfections" would vary to match each patient's predominant concerns. Though similar in form, the treatments' content differed to capture each patient's idiosyncratic thoughts, feelings, and actions. For the residents, appreciating patients' distinctive illness experiences meant developing a new framework for connecting diagnoses, symptoms, and interventions.

To borrow a phrase I heard frequently in the field, the residents had to learn that "every patient is different" and that, more than understanding what diagnoses patients shared, the task was to understand the unique ways in which they suffered.[3] This was the only way to craft treatments that worked. "There's this perception [that] CBT is really manualized, and it is to some extent," Jackie, an experienced psychologist specializing in CBT, told me. "But it's not," she asserted. "With anxiety disorders," Jackie's area of expertise, "it's all about trying to develop an exposure program that really gets to the core of the person's anxiety." With clients, she explained, she's "trying to figure out: 'Can I put myself in your head and figure out what situations would make you anxious?'" Though CBT is formulaic, Jackie made clear that the process of its application was creative and "idiosyncratic." She had to "put" herself into patients' "heads" to figure out their specific triggers and experiences. To accomplish this feat, the residents would have to accept that knowledge of diagnoses or symptoms would be insufficient.

DSM Diagnoses as Obstacles to Psychodynamic Understanding

It was in psychodynamic psychotherapy that the loss of categorical thinking took its most acute form. During one October meeting of the psychodynamic core class, Terry and Patricia, the psychoanalysts who ran the rotation, asked the residents whether they talked with their patients about their sexual lives. The residents' approach was summed up by Cedric (PGY-3): they did so to "try to identify a pathology to it, [the patient's] pathology, and to see how that relates to the axes and diagnoses." Cedric was referencing the five axes and more than three hundred diagnoses of the DSM-IV-TR, the version of the DSM current at the time of my fieldwork (described in chapter 2). Terry responded:

> I think you're raising an interesting point [about] the differences between thinking psychodynamically and psychiatrically—that sometimes is used in a pejorative way by [psycho]analysts. . . . In a psychiatric eval, you look at the DSM, a disease model of pathology, what is wrong with the person? A psychodynamic diagnosis is aimed at understanding who the person is. . . . You're not looking at a dimensional understanding of the person, but you want to understand "how does this person function?" But they're different diagnostic tasks.

I had heard Terry and the other psychoanalysts I spoke with make versions of this comment numerous times. Psychoanalysis and psychodynamic psychotherapy had, in their telling, a radically distinct goal compared with biological psychiatry. For the residents, Terry's explanation encapsulated the dilemmas of switching epistemic lenses. Whereas biopsychiatry required them to focus on patients' "pathology," psychodynamic psychotherapy called on them to understand "who the person is," as Terry put it. The DSM would be useless, even detrimental, as they sought to get to know their patients. To arrive at a "psychodynamic diagnosis," they would have to do nothing less than unravel the ways in which the patient "functions" as a person in the world. Accomplishing these distinct "diagnostic tasks" presented the early psychiatrists with antithetical models of doctoring.

I had begun to understand what doctoring psychodynamically would mean during my initial visits to the rotation, more than a year earlier. I first came to Shorewood to observe three "intake" interviews that Terry conducted with a patient to help familiarize the residents with the psychodynamic approach. The patient was Rob, a man in his late twenties who had come to the clinic complaining of depression caused, in his telling, by ongoing struggles finishing his graduate work. Accustomed to intake interviews that focused on the patient's history of the illness, symptoms, and diagnosis, the residents wanted to hear Terry discuss his own, quite different technique. During one postsession debriefing conversation, Zoli, a PGY-3 at the time, asked:

> *Zoli (PGY-3)*: This goes along with our [previous] discussion about [medical versus psychodynamic] models. . . . You spent some time going over the [patient's] substance use history but less time going over the mood disorder. Can you talk about your decision not to pursue that?
> *Terry (Instructor)*: I use sessions to go where the feelings go, [to] go with the affect.

Zoli was puzzled by Terry's use of some diagnostic questions but not others. Substance abuse, I would later learn, is thought to interfere with and even be made worse by the kind of intensive self-reflection required in long-term psychodynamic therapy. In contrast, a DSM-informed understanding of Rob's mood-related illness was not, Terry made clear, necessary for moving forward with psychodynamic treatment. Though Terry would go on to ask Rob some questions related to a major depression diagnosis in the following session, even those focused on Rob's past experiences with the illness and thus did not amount to a formal diagnostic interview. In going "with the affect," Terry was trying to understand how his patient "functioned" as a "person."

During the conversations that followed, I was surprised to find that, despite the wealth of information Rob had shared about himself, both Terry and the residents characterized their understanding of him as "superficial." Yet I would later learn that their agreement was cursory. Though they had arrived at the same conclusion, their logics differed, pitting the experienced psychoanalyst's pursuit of unconscious conflicts against the psychiatrists' search for diagnostic clarity. Terry thought that although Rob had offered many interesting leads (an absent father, a troubled early psychoanalysis, an extended hospitalization), he did not reveal much of his emotional life. For their part, the residents could not identify Rob's diagnosis, nor did they have a clear picture of his symptoms and the history of his illness. The residents found it difficult to let go of the professional utility and security of the DSM. Through symptoms, they could understand and treat patients' diseases, track the progress of treatment, communicate with other medical professionals, and fulfill their bureaucratic duties. In psychodynamic psychotherapy, they learned that symptoms were only a flawed and narrow lens into patients' inner lives.

To be clear, psychodynamic clinicians did not eschew the DSM altogether. Ronald, an experienced psychoanalyst who served as a supervisor to some of the residents in the program, told me, "I use [the DSM] to convince an insurance company [*laughs*] . . . that the patient has some difficulties that are [treatable]." Though a good tool for getting paid, the DSM fell epistemically short in Ronald's view: "I don't find its logic that helpful in the kind of work that I do." This stance was common among the psychodynamic psychotherapists and psychoanalysts with whom I spoke. For them, the DSM was a tool with which they could legitimate and support their work. Substantively, it did little to help them understand patients' problems. This limitation was troubling for the residents: they had developed their professional knowledge of what patients suffer from by memorizing DSM symptoms and categories. Its worthlessness in psychodynamic psychotherapy challenged their expectations about how to doctor.

In their search for epistemic anchors, the residents hoped that psychoanalytic theory might offer them an alternative to the DSM. Instead, they were repeatedly told that attempting to craft a general explanation for patients' problems was less important than seeking to understand their particular experiences. The lesson became clear during conversations about child development and its reverberations into adulthood. Nathan (PGY-3) asked what "trajectory" would be expected "if someone who is ten [years old] gets emotionally abused." Instead of offering conceptual clarity, Terry encouraged the residents to think about patients' idiosyncrasies: "There's a very interesting concept of multifinality, which means that the same insult can present in a myriad [of] ways, depending on the person. And multideterminacy [means that] quite different insults can lead to the same presentation. . . . In a sense, each patient needs to be taken at face value."

In psychodynamic therapy, taking each patient "at face value" meant that every person's path to illness is unique and must be understood as such. Even as psychoanalytic theories may offer ways to conceptualize patients' experiences, understanding the nuances of such experiences took precedence. In fact, Terry proposed, the residents ought to be prepared for the unexpected. They could not assume to find a causal arrow connecting an "insult," a troubling early experience, with the same set of symptoms in different patients. Nor should they be surprised if distinct problems result in similar symptoms. All the residents could do, and the best they could do, is understand each patient's life history and relationships. Only then could they arrive at a psychodynamic understanding of the unique unconscious troubles animating the person sitting across from them. But this was still far from the junior residents' epistemic imaginaries. Without the use of symptoms and diagnoses, and with little knowledge of the psychoanalytic canon, the residents were intellectually unmoored.

UNSETTLING EPISTEMIC AUTHORITY

Doctors exercise epistemic authority over patients' problems by interpreting them through the lenses of diagnosis and treatment.[4] In much of medicine, such authority is partly facilitated by technologies, such as scans and tests, that make the body visible. In mental health, despite advancements in pharmacogenomics and neuroscience, psychiatrists and other professionals have yet to find a diagnostic test that can validly and reliably identify mental illnesses.[5] This means that, in practical terms, clinicians must rely largely on observations of patients' behaviors and, more prevalently, on patients' own reports about their experiences. In this context, mental health practice is oriented toward the management of doubt: Is the patient fully revealing his suffering? Is she disclosing the frequency with which she contemplates suicide? Is he really hearing voices and accurately reporting their content? Did they follow treatment as prescribed and are they being honest about other chemical substances they are consuming? These and myriad other questions come up when practitioners try to make sense of their patients' troubles. While doubts about patients' reports are not unusual in medicine, they are constitutive of working in mental health.[6]

In biopsychiatry, the residents learn to manage these sources of doubt by privileging their own observations of patients' behavior and demeanor and by relying on diagnostic questionnaires and targeted inquiries about drug effects.[7] And while none of these strategies eliminate the mediating role of patients' stories, they do offer the residents—and psychiatrists more broadly—a way to achieve a modicum of what historian Ted Porter called "mechanical objectivity," the objectivity associated with measurement and observability.[8] In turn, these same tools signal psychiatrists' epistemic authority, granting them interpretative power over patients' experiences.

In psychotherapy, the residents have less epistemic control. Here, the stories that patients share about themselves and their relationships are the principal data the residents must work with and make sense of. In turn, the veracity, accuracy, and completeness of patients' accounts become catalysts for the residents' skepticism, particularly early in their psychotherapy training. In psychodynamic psychotherapy they learn that the roots of patients' problems are out of their awareness, residing in the unconscious. Patients are by definition unable to identify and reveal these forces unless they engage in the self-reflective work of psychotherapy. For its part, CBT attributes patients' troubles to behaviors and automatic thoughts that are conscious and can be accessed through careful guidance and questioning from the therapist. Yet even here, as I show next, patients are not always able or willing to identify the specific actions or thoughts that cause their ill feelings. Unsurprisingly, the residents find the psychotherapies'—and thus their own—reliance on patients disquieting.

Searching for Complete and Accurate Accounts in CBT

In CBT, just as in biopsychiatry, the residents counted on patients' true and accurate accounts of their illness experiences to make sense of their suffering and offer appropriate interventions. Yet whereas pharmacology appointments entailed relatively brief discussions of symptoms and drug effects, CBT required the residents to become adept at accessing patients' thoughts, feelings, and behaviors in greater depth. But, the residents would find, patients were seldom willing or able to collaborate in this project of self-knowledge.

Early in the CBT for anxiety rotation, one of the social work fellows presented the case of a woman who had failed to complete her homework exercises despite rating them relatively painless on a "subjective units of distress scale" (SUDS). This led Jeremy, the instructor, to surmise, "My gut tells me that she's probably a little afraid, a little scared." Ely (PGY-3) agreed: "I'm guessing that maybe her 50s and 60s [scores on the SUDS scale] are more like 70s and 80s." Ely was not surprised that a patient would downplay or, as mental health practitioners sometimes put it, underreport, her distress.

Anticipating such difficulties, CBT clinicians and biopsychiatrists rely on "inscriptive" tools—namely, standardized forms—intended to capture a more accurate picture of patients' suffering.[9] The residents were familiar with some of these tools, particularly the diagnostic forms commonly used to classify patients' symptoms. The forms offer mental health clinicians a way to track, measure, and compare patients' states over time. The forms are material representations of doctors' epistemic authority, interpellating patients into particular kinds of disclosure and shaping their narratives about their experiences.[10] For the residents and their colleagues, they function as professional aids, doing some of the work of untangling and distilling patients' mental and emotional lives into those components deemed essential in CBT and pharmacology.

When Robert, the instructor in CBT for depression, introduced the residents to specific forms during the first meeting of his rotation, he explained about one of them:

A daily mood record, on the left side it's got their mood score from 0 to 10 and on the other side it has a number of pleasant activities. . . . You don't have to initially include that piece, but if you look at this as a daily mood record, you can have people do this before they go to bed . . . [and] you can go over it with them [in session] looking for significant ups and downs. . . . It also can be a corrective for a person's thinking that "I always feel the same," that there's no fluctuation, by seeing that there's some change.

When patients have been depressed for some time, they can misrecognize and thus misreport their own moods. A "daily mood record" can help both patient and therapist gain a more accurate understanding of the patient's states. The form also facilitates access to the patient's inner life and symptoms, turning them into actionable CBT data. The residents, akin to CBT clinicians and other mental health practitioners, relied on such forms to gain knowledge of patients' illness experiences. The forms ease the burden of access and mitigate issues of trust and accuracy: whereas patients cannot be trusted to accurately capture "fluctuations" in their moods, forms can. Crucially, the forms allowed the residents to maintain their epistemic authority, bestowing a sense of objectivity on their work and shoring up their professional identities as physicians.

Yet these inscriptive tools did not solve all the problems associated with constructing a truthful and accurate picture of patients' suffering. Sonora's experience treating Sam was emblematic in this respect. Her setbacks made clear that implementing CBT depended on a diagnosis as much as it did on knowing the thoughts, feelings, and behaviors that animated Sam's symptoms. About a month into their meetings, Sonora found herself in the thick of uncertainty and frustration. As Sam steadfastly withheld access to his worries, and with no clear diagnosis to rely on, the group had to piece together a picture of what may have been troubling him. The situation had made a straightforward CBT treatment nearly impossible.

During one especially fraught session, Sonora asked Sam, "So what are the bothersome thoughts . . . you said that your thoughts go places you don't want them to, so what are they?" She reiterated the importance of identifying his specific thoughts to begin treatment: "You know we haven't been really doing CBT, because we don't really know where to focus." Sam reluctantly admitted to having thoughts about "sex, being into people, lying to someone." Sonora insisted:

> *Sonora (PGY-4)*: So what is the actual thought?
> *Sam (Patient)*: Nothing in particular, just a broad range of me not being perfect . . .
> *Sonora*: I'm asking you because CBT is very specific. So we need to get to very specific thoughts about sex.
> *Sam*: Well, they always seem to change, all of them . . . I don't know if there is one that reoccurs . . . But it just bothers me that they're there.

Sam's inability or, as the team came to believe, unwillingness, to be more "specific" about his troubles, made his suffering inaccessible and, from the standpoint of CBT, untreatable. Sam's case was "hard," Sonora told her colleagues, because, as she put it, "it's so freaking abstract." Such "abstractness" is anathema to CBT interventions. In a pharmacology appointment, Sonora would have already prescribed a medication and simply focused on assessing how it affected Sam's ongoing symptoms (another resident at the clinic was doing just that with him). In CBT, she could hardly move forward without a detailed understanding of the thoughts that crossed Sam's mind when he was most distressed. No forms and questionnaires could help with an unwilling patient.

Making Sense of Patients' Incomplete Stories in Psychodynamic Psychotherapy

Accepting their dependence on patients fit uneasily with the residents' existing expectations about how patients and doctors communicate and what they each must do in a medical encounter. This particular source of friction was especially pronounced when the residents doubted the veracity or completeness of their patients' accounts, something that happened more frequently than I expected. During a conversation in the psychodynamic group, Russ (PGY-4) declared:

> *Russ (PGY-4)*: We give recommendations for treatment based on what the patient is telling us!
>
> *Terry (Instructor)*: It has to be [that way], but it's not only on that, that's why they call you an expert . . .
>
> *Russ*: We're basing treatment on what we're being told and who knows if what we're being told is true or complete! I have a specific example where I had a patient tell me this week that there's a lot of stuff that he hadn't told me about, and that would have changed how I would have approached his treatment!

Russ's predicament was only unusual in the patient's honesty. Weeks away from their final session together, the resident had learned that his patient had been less than forthcoming about his life. The resident's indignant tone revealed his frustration. His patient's last-minute disclosure had placed into question their entire psychotherapeutic treatment. It had also made plain the limitations the residents had to confront while doing therapy. Russ's experience brought forth in the starkest possible light their dependence on patients. Despite Terry's assurance that Russ and his colleagues could count on their budding status as "experts" to manage this dilemma, patients' inability or, as was the case here, unwillingness to disclose fueled the residents' skepticism toward the very possibility of successful psychotherapy.

Terry sought to offer the residents a distinct orientation toward matters of truth and accuracy in psychodynamic psychotherapy. He encouraged them to cultivate their curiosity, even in the disheartening circumstances Russ described: "It's best to wonder, why is this information coming out *now*, what prompted the patient to tell me this *now*?" The patient, Terry proposed, was worried about the end of therapy and, in sharing his nondisclosure, signaled a latent wish to prolong the therapeutic relationship. Rather than a treatment debacle, the experienced psychoanalyst suggested, Russ should take the patient's confession as a sign of his therapeutic skill. The resident had approached his patient's disclosure with a biopsychiatric lens. In psychodynamic psychotherapy, epistemic authority took on new meaning.

Terry's suggestion was more than practicable advice for the frustrated resident. It also hinted at a different approach to doctoring. Psychodynamic psychotherapy challenged the notion, central to medical practice, that patients needed to report their illnesses truthfully and accurately so that their physicians can arrive at an appropriate diagnosis and prescribe an appropriate treatment. In psychodynamic psychotherapy, Terry made clear, curiosity rather than skepticism would help the residents better understand their patients, even when the patients seemed poised to disclose little. Practically, an inquisitive stance, coupled with patience, would be the residents' best tool. But this doctoring approach ran counter to the directive authority the residents had internalized as medication prescribers.

This discussion should not be taken to mean that psychodynamic psychotherapists expected their patients to lie or that they accepted untruths as facts. Rather, given their focus on unconscious dynamics, truth has to be understood differently—less as a matter of historical fact and more as a matter of meaning. The residents wanted to get their patients' stories right, but, as Lucas (PGY-4), pointed out, "the danger is that, just because something [a patient said] sounds plausible, it doesn't mean it's true." Terry summed up the conundrum as a question: "Is the veridicality of the patient's story as important as the fact that the patient *has* a story?" This "unresolved controversy" in the psychoanalytic "literature," as Terry described it, left some residents doubtful. But, the further along they were in their psychotherapy training, the more likely they were to echo a psychodynamic perspective. Jake (PGY-4) summed up the discussion by proposing that when "someone tells you what happened in their life at [age] five," they are signaling something that is important to their sense of self, "regardless [of] whether it's true or not." Terry agreed: "If it helps [the patient] figure out something that's going on in their life, that's what it's about." The residents would have to accept the psychodynamic commitment to, as Terry put it, take patients "at face value" and understand who they are rather than simply what symptoms ail them.

The residents' experiences, whether in psychodynamic psychotherapy or in CBT, pointed to a fundamental conundrum: could they conduct therapy without patients' truthful, complete, and accurate disclosures? After all, their own ability to diagnose and treat seemed to depend on precisely such accounts. But patients have difficult relationships with their mental illnesses, more so because of shame, fear, and stigma.[11] It is thus not surprising that the residents frequently ran into barriers as they sought to gain a psychotherapeutic understanding of their patients' problems. And although their more experienced instructors and supervisors could prepare them for such challenges, the residents had yet to acquire the clinical experience necessary to turn problems into psychotherapeutic opportunities. What these experiences did accomplish was to further unmoor the residents' biopsychiatric assumptions and their sense of epistemic authority. In turn, confronting a different doctoring mandate opened the door for skepticism toward the very possibility of conducting psychotherapy.

Professional Friction

The residents' expectations about what it means to be a psychiatrist were upended not only epistemically but also professionally. They entered psychotherapy training just as they anticipated a move, in their third postgraduate year, to a more autonomous status. The residents had spent years being novices, first as medical students, then as interns, and finally as residents on psychiatric units. Their transition to the clinic entailed treating patients in individual offices and signaled greater independence. Psychotherapy training presented them with the paradoxes of becoming novices anew. Their dilemmas converged on maintaining authoritative personas in the context of subordinate relationships with psychotherapy instructors and individual supervisors. In the following pages, I highlight two sources of professional friction as they manifested themselves in relationships between residents and their superiors in psychotherapy: first, the challenges of becoming novices and managing oversight, and second, the struggle for professional self-determination in contexts organized around fostering self-reflexivity through self-work.

BEING COMPELLED INTO PSYCHOTHERAPEUTIC NOVICEHOOD

Psychotherapy instructors were aware of the residents' contradictory positions and sought to implement and communicate their expectations while recognizing their status as budding professionals. For example, all instructors firmly believed that the residents would learn talk and behavioral interventions best if they employed them during actual treatments with patients. And while the residents were required to do so in psychodynamic psychotherapy, Terry and Patricia—the psychodynamic instructors—could not compel them to take on the number of patients nor see them with the frequency that the experienced analysts saw fit. For their part, cognitive and behavioral instructors expected but did not require the residents to conduct treatments with their particular approach. Nevertheless, this expectation was evident in the common practice of starting every meeting by inviting the residents to discuss their conundrums implementing therapeutic techniques with their patients. The invitation implicitly communicated to the novice therapists that they ought to put CBT and other approaches into practice even with patients whom they treated pharmacologically.

Yet even when the residents did work with patients psychotherapeutically, their instructors infrequently had opportunities to observe them doing so. On the few occasions when this happened in CBT training, the residents' inexperience showed, a persistent reminder of their therapeutic novicehood. Whether they relied on pagers to receive practical hints from instructors watching from behind a one-way mirror or conducted sessions alongside them, the residents could seem more like intermediaries between instructors and patients, rather than their patients' main doctors. A message received too late or awkwardly implemented in the session, or a question better delivered by the instructor, could highlight rather than smooth over the resident's inexperience. And whereas some appreciated the opportunity of being observed and given direct feedback, others chafed at the possibility and sought to avoid it. It was only a reminder of their contradictory roles as professional novices.

With few opportunities for direct observation, instructors devised alternative means for compelling the residents to do some of the work of novicehood. All psychotherapy rotations revolved around clinical case presentations and discussions in which residents were expected to talk about their psychotherapeutic treatment conundrums. These forms of instruction are commonplace in medical training, and the residents had much experience navigating them. Yet their experience was in biopsychiatry, and, as I will show in chapters 5 and 6, their skills did not translate neatly into the psychotherapy setting. Whether they failed to describe the contexts in which a patient's symptoms became acute or the thoughts that seemed to animate those symptoms, or focused on a patient's medical history rather than their life and relationships, the residents' loss of professional anchors showed. No longer opportunities for showcasing their mastery of an epistemic domain and their growing professional status, case presentations and discussions by junior residents served as another reminder of their positions as psychotherapy novices.

In addition to case discussions and presentations, CBT instructors also relied on role-play and homework to instruct and assess the residents. Role-play, a topic I return to in chapter 5, compelled the residents to showcase their CBT abilities—or, as was the case, inabilities—by taking on parts as therapists or patients and practicing particular techniques. Instructors used role-play to model therapeutic interactions, leading their partners through the intricacies of identifying patients' thoughts and feelings, or implementing specific techniques. But, more than a tool of instruction, role-play was also, in only implicitly, a conduit of supervision, affording CBT instructors a means to assess the residents' skills.

Finally, the residents, akin to patients, also had to complete "homework." Nora, the social worker who ran the dialectical behavioral therapy

(DBT) rotation, made clear early on that everyone, including me, would have to use DBT tools and skills in our work and everyday lives. She began every meeting by asking each of us what we had accomplished with DBT and ended every discussion by having us choose a technique or principle to implement. Nora made it clear that nobody was forced to discuss their conundrums with the group nor disclose anything "embarrassing," as one resident worried they might. Nevertheless, over the six months we saw one another, every day started with a discussion of our homework.

For her part, Nora was cognizant of the residents' role contradictions. During one meeting halfway through the rotation, she asked them whether they found it "demeaning to be asked to do homework." She continued, "I want to know with doctors, as prescribers, is it off-putting to talk about homework? I bring this up because [during] the last [rotation] people had a complaint about it." At times, the residents actively resisted their new roles: they "complained" about their duties, questioned instructors' approaches, and pushed against the new authority structures they entered. That day, Sawyer (PGY-4) admitted, "I guess my first reaction with any kind of homework is, ugh!" But, he continued, "when you think about it, it forces you to keep DBT in mind all the time." Sawyer's response was emblematic of the friction he and his colleagues faced: though wary of being treated like novices, they knew that they could only learn psychotherapy by submitting to the demands of the role.

The residents' dilemmas as professional novices were even more pronounced in psychodynamic instruction. The program required them to meet once a week with a psychoanalyst to discuss the psychodynamic psychotherapy treatments they conducted at the clinic. Such meetings revolved around the residents' "process notes," a ubiquitous technique of supervision in this epistemic community. At their most basic, such notes contain transcripts, rendered from memory, of therapy sessions. Ideally, they would convey subtler and more encompassing information about therapeutic interactions. Turner (PGY-3) explained that "the concept of a process note is that you're assuming everything in the room has meaning and not leaving anything out that you could actually remember." Such detailed accounting of therapeutic interactions can make for rich conversations about therapy sessions. Producing them was no small feat, adding to the residents' existing temporal burden. Terry admitted that process notes are "very taxing to do," but, he urged, "they can be very useful" by yielding "data to use in pattern recognition."

Process notes, like role-play, serve as tools of both training and oversight. Early in the residents' therapeutic training, they could reveal their taken-for-granted doctoring practices, giving supervisors grounds for intervention. Hugh, an experienced psychoanalyst who supervised some of the residents in the program, told me about a trainee who had arrived to one of their initial meetings with "an evaluation of a patient done on the basis of the DSM-IV model." The resident, Hugh told me, "had a lot of data about the patient, but it was not very meaningful." Age, a history of abuse, colleges, marriages, siblings, and physical symptoms were all described in neat, medical fashion. Hugh encouraged the resident to approach the patient in a more open-ended way. But, during their next meeting, another set of process notes revealed that the resident had, the psychoanalyst exclaimed, done "more of the same!"

Hugh encouraged the resident to simply "have a chat with the person, you know, about her life, like you were sitting at the bar." This time, new process notes showed the strategy had worked: "And all of a sudden, a whole new world opened up of this person's marital difficulties, her children, her [. . .] troubles with her parents, a potential mistreatment as a young person." Significantly, the resident was no longer speaking the language of biological psychiatry: they had inhabited a psychodynamic role and begun to understand the patient as a person. With the aid of process notes, Hugh and his colleagues could compel the residents into the role of trainee and steer them toward psychodynamic doctoring practices.

As productive as it could be, this model of supervision proved troubling, especially for junior residents. A discussion in the psychodynamic meeting revealed some of their concerns:

> *Julian (PGY-3)*: When we get new patients here [at the clinic] there's always an attendant who lays eyes on the patient . . . But with our psychodynamics, our supervisors don't see our patients . . . I thought it would be helpful for me to record a session and bring it into the supervision, but my supervisor resisted that . . .
>
> *Zaheed (PGY-3)*: I oftentimes feel like I'm not conveying the patient . . . it would be nice to have a recording . . . I try to stay faithful to what we each said, but sometimes I'm not able to convey the flavor or the tone of the session . . .

Julian and Zaheed voiced a common source of strain among the residents: how can a supervisor make appropriate treatment recommendations when they never observe the residents interacting with their patients? The question hinted at the residents' expectations of what their training should look like. Having a more experienced doctor "lay eyes on the patient" is a central element of medical education—and assuages novices' anxieties. In psychodynamic supervision, even as they stayed "faithful" to the words exchanged in session, the residents couldn't help but feel that they fell short of fully capturing "the flavor or the tone of the session," as Zaheed put it. The residents were troubled by the interpretive distance between supervisor and treatment and by what this distance meant for their own professional positions.

While these early PGY-3s worried about their ability to accurately "convey" therapeutic interactions to their supervisors, Andrea (PGY-4), an advanced resident, offered a contrasting perspective. "If I'm missing something in the patient," she explained with confidence, "that's what I'm working with." Her stance revealed the effects of two years of training in psychodynamic psychotherapy and her accumulated competence in the approach. The residents, Andrea asserted, are always basing their interventions on their own understanding of the patient and their treatment. As such, the fact that supervisors have access to nothing other than their reports was unproblematic. Andrea's junior colleagues had yet to embrace this stance. They were accustomed to assuming that accuracy, rather than meaning, would govern their and their supervisors' treatment decisions. They had also yet to submit to the demands of being psychotherapy trainees.

Individual supervision made clear the contradictions embedded in the residents' roles. Julian and Zaheed were not simply worried about how well their supervisors could understand their patients. Fundamentally, if only implicitly, they were also questioning the bases of their supervisors' authority. The residents felt this friction most acutely when they disagreed with their supervisors' treatment suggestions. "I'm the therapist for this patient," Octavia (PGY-3) told Ely (PGY-4) indignantly before the start of one psychotherapy rotation. "But," she continued, "after multiple discussions with my psychodynamic supervisor, she felt that she wanted to stick to psychodynamic [therapy] for now." Instead, Octavia asserted, "I really think that [my patient] needs DBT!" "She comes in one time and she's really angry, and she's really trying to control it," Octavia offered by way of justification. "Or she's coming in and crying uncontrollably!"

Ely, the more senior resident, sought to assuage his junior colleague's concerns and offer some assurance: "Remember that your supervisor is an adviser, not the boss." He continued, "So if you have someone who needs a more acute intervention, you need to go and talk to many other people, like the attending [psychiatrist]." Ultimately, however, Octavia would decide on the course of treatment. "Go with the advice that you think is best for the patient," Ely concluded. In a field where each intervention can marshal its own evidence of efficacy, residents have few uncontested tools at their disposal when making difficult decisions about treatment, especially when such decisions go against a supervisor's advice.[12] Individual supervisors might suggest, or even insist on, divergent courses of action. Octavia felt the precariousness of her authority, despite being "the therapist for [her] patient." She tried to establish her budding autonomy by appeal to her clinical knowledge: she, not her supervisor, was the one in the room with the patient, observing and experiencing her demeanor and emotions. She was thus best positioned to know what kind of psychotherapy her patient needed.

Octavia's assertions hinted at a common strategy the residents employed when faced with professional friction; namely, appealing to clinical experience. To establish their knowledge and distance themselves from the status of novices, the residents claimed to know their patients best: the range of their symptoms, the depth of their despair, what they could and could not accomplish in treatment. Such claims, however, became muddled when confronted with a supervisor's insistence on a divergent course of action, an insistence based on their own clinical experience. These instances crystallized the residents' contradictory positions as novices and professionals. They also triggered their skepticism toward psychotherapy training.

RECKONING WITH THE DEMANDS OF
SELF-REFLEXIVITY IN PSYCHOTHERAPY

Psychotherapy training posed the residents with an additional challenge: to achieve competence, they had to develop self-reflexivity. Their instructors sought to foster this skill through group and individual conversations, homework exercises, or role-play. For the residents, this was an unanticipated dimension of doctoring, one that they had not been encouraged to cultivate in their earlier training. In psychotherapy, the process was rife with friction, subverting their ideas about professional detachment and threatening their sense of authority.

These dynamics were especially pronounced in the residents' interactions with their psychoanalytic supervisors. Psychodynamic psychotherapy considers the therapeutic relationship to be an essential platform for uncovering and addressing patients' unconscious conflicts; the therapist's actions—motivated by conscious and unconscious forces—are constitutive of it. In supervision, Terry explained, this would mean that "the material that we're working with is our interaction with the patient." Such interactions, psychoanalysts know well, are shaped both by the person receiving care and by the one offering it. Practically, this meant that the residents had to understand the dynamics of treatment interactions by examining not only their patients' inner lives but also their own. Much of this knowledge came about in individual supervision, sometimes to the residents' dismay. Their ambivalence about the supervisory dynamics created in the process became evident during an end-of-year conversation in the psychodynamic rotation:

> *Zoli (PGY-4)*: One of the things that we started talking about was the hetero-geneity of supervision, and in that Gabbard book there was a beginning chapter about supervision, and I thought that was really helpful, like, for example, that you're not a patient . . .
>
> *Terry (Instructor)*: Supervision becomes psychotherapy?
>
> *Zoli*: Either that or sometimes the supervisor gives more career or personal advice that is not solicited by the resident . . .
>
> *Terry*: Within supervision it's entirely legit [for the supervisor] to say, "It appears that some personal things of yours are interfering with the treat-ment, so you need to find a way to deal with that." . . . It's a complicated area but your point is well taken . . .
>
> *Patricia (Instructor)*: What isn't OK [is] to go into those personal issues, that would not be appropriate . . .
>
> *Alayna (PGY-3)*: But in a way it's helpful . . .
>
> *Jason (PGY-4)*: Yes it is . . .

Becoming akin to a patient in psychoanalytic supervision only height-ened the professional friction the residents experienced as novices in psy-chotherapy. Zoli was troubled by supervisors who offered "advice" on personal and professional matters that was "not solicited." The residents struggled with the heightened power imbalance this could introduce in the psychodynamic supervisory relationship. Their supervisors could tell them how to treat their patients even as they had never observed them actually interact. They could point out the residents' missteps, highlighting their novice ignorance. And, more troublingly, they at times traced the roots of such missteps to the residents' own inner lives. This was not the pro-fessional distance that the residents had been accustomed to during their biopsychiatric training. And while some residents found such attention useful, as Alayna (PGY-3) and Jason (PGY-4) made clear, others chafed at this dimension of supervision.

Nevertheless, even as they sought to assume some control over their roles in supervision, the residents did eventually submit to the demand for self-reflexivity in psychodynamic training. This became clearer during a group discussion:

> *Terry (Instructor)*: That brings up the question about the boundaries of supervision. . . . How do you not go into therapy?
>
> *Jake (PGY-4) [asking Terry]*: How do you not become the therapist for the consultee?

Vinit (PGY-4): How much does the supervisor need to be a therapist in order to understand the case presented, which is very filtered? I'm wondering, thinking of our own supervision, because none of us have been in analysis [*laughter in the room, someone comments that he doesn't know that*[13]] . . . and I spend a lot of time thinking about why I present the case the way I do . . .

Lucas (PGY-3): You could be fortunate enough to have an omniscient supervisor like me and he can figure out what's missing from that presentation . . . I'm still looking for the bug in my office!

Russ (PGY-4): The reality is that data is not just data. . . . I can describe the facts, but how I describe them and my tone of voice matter too.

The advanced residents were acutely aware that their professional performances in supervision were as much objects of analysis as patients' own words. But, rather than chafing against this dimension of novicehood, they embraced it. For Vinit (PGY-4), self-reflexivity, developed during psychodynamic training, meant spending "a lot of time thinking about why" he presents "the case the way" he does. The residents' earlier education in biopsychiatry had neither fostered nor required such self-awareness. Psychodynamic psychotherapy demanded it, and individual supervision was one of its main conduits. For the residents, this meant submitting to the distinct demands of being a novice in psychotherapy—whether by learning new approaches or by reflecting on their doctoring and personal selves.

Such self-awareness was not unique to psychodynamic therapy, though it did take a particular form here. Indeed, as I show in chapter 5, "homework" and "role-play" in CBT and DBT were intended to teach residents therapeutic techniques by compelling them to work on themselves. And while becoming more self-reflexive was a welcomed dimension of learning psychotherapy, the process was rife with professional friction. For the residents, learning psychotherapy was thus not simply about being pegged as novices even as they were already doctors. It was also about letting go of some of the professional remove they had come to associate with being a doctor and unwittingly becoming akin to patients, working on themselves with the therapeutic tools they were learning. Though they chafed at this development, with time, as I show in later chapters, this self-reflexivity would become an essential ingredient in their transition from skepticism to competence.

Conclusion

Professional socialization introduces novices to new ways of seeing the world and their place in it. The residents at Shorewood had been socialized to "recognize" mental illness biopsychiatrically during medical school, internship, and their time working with hospitalized patients. In this perspective, problems of behavior, thinking, or feeling constitute symptoms, the outward manifestations of patients' brain diseases. In turn, symptoms are targets of treatment and measures of its success. Psychotherapy challenged the residents to shift their perspective. While CBT afforded them greater epistemic stability with its emphasis on symptoms and diagnoses, it also posed them new challenges. To put CBT tools and skills into practice, the residents had to discern patients' idiosyncratic constellations of thoughts, feelings, and behaviors. In psychodynamic psychotherapy, symptoms are merely the superficial manifestations of patients' unconscious conflicts, and the residents had to learn to think beyond them, focusing instead on patients' personal histories and relationships.

The conflicting assumptions and practices of biopsychiatric, psychodynamic, and cognitive behavioral approaches gave rise to the epistemic friction that defined the residents' training in psychotherapy. Reconfiguring their knowledge into psychotherapeutic frameworks required them to let go of psychiatric diagnosis even as they had become skilled diagnosticians, grapple with understanding how "every patient is different" even as patients seemed to fit into the same disease categories, and wrestle with a distinct orientation toward their very object of knowledge; namely, patients' inner lives. Part of what made the loss of diagnosis so destabilizing was the loss of rules. One of the key insights that studies of professional socialization have offered us is that, early in their training, novices rely on rules to learn and practice a new craft.[14] Expertise comes about only when such rules become internalized and are treated more like guidelines and less like decrees.[15] For the residents, a focus on symptoms and diagnoses was both institutionally required and epistemically expeditious.[16] This focus should not be taken to mean that the residents viewed DSM diagnoses as perfect reflections of their patients' suffering, however. Their approach, as I pointed out in chapter 2 and as other social scientists have shown, was more pragmatic: slotting patients into broad categories such as depression or anxiety was secondary to understanding their symptoms but still provided a useful starting point for figuring out a treatment path.[17]

More than serving epistemic function, classifying patients' illnesses through the lens of symptoms and diagnoses is an important mark of professional status. Science and technology scholars have shown that professionals rely on systems of classification and standardization to shore up their claims to expertise and authority.[18] For the residents, losing that foundation, even partially as in CBT, was thus not only epistemically destabilizing, it also reverberated into their very sense of themselves as professionals. As biopsychiatrists, they could rely on observational data and diagnostic forms and questionnaires to do the work of doctoring: construct a medical history, assign a diagnosis, treat. This same approach was ill suited for getting into patients' "heads," to paraphrase Jackie, the experienced CBT practitioner. The residents' experiences with patients' concealments—whether intentional or not—affirmed their dependence on the very people they were trying to help. It brought into relief their mediated expertise and highlighted their fragile epistemic authority.

Entering psychotherapeutic training unmoored not only the residents' epistemic anchors but also their professional identities. The move to the clinic from the hospital had come with the promise of greater independence. Being able to meet with patients in their own offices was not simply a signal of the relative health of those patients but also a mark of the residents' own growing autonomy. In these spaces, the residents were relatively insulated from the gaze of senior psychiatrists and did what they knew best: pharmacology. In psychotherapy, they struggled to reconcile this burgeoning professional authority with the constraints of their beginner status. The paradox of being directed in a treatment that they were seldom or, as was the case in psychodynamic psychotherapy, never directly observed doing provoked the residents' frustration and, at times, skepticism. This skepticism became especially problematic when supervisors' suggestions targeted not only their therapeutic knowledge but also their ability to tune into their inner lives. Professional work could quickly become personal, giving rise to uneasy role contradictions.

The residents' early forays into psychotherapy training were thus marked by a heightened sense of epistemic and professional friction. Whether they had to set aside their biopsychiatric knowledge, get to know their patients in deeper and more personal ways, or reconsider their expectations about truth and accuracy in treatment, the residents had to rethink their assumptions about mental illness and its care. They also had to navigate the conundrums of being at once novices and professionals. Their doctoring expectations were unmoored. Aware of their contradictory positions, their instructors sought to offer them new anchors, new ways to think about themselves and their patients. I turn next to their strategies for making psychotherapy intelligible and credible to their skeptical audience.

4 * Psychotherapy Instructors

Terry, the experienced psychiatrist and psychoanalyst who co-led the psychodynamic rotation, was an enthusiastic proponent of the approach. One early morning in March, I joined him for an introductory lecture to a cohort of residents in their second postgraduate year (PGY-2). The meeting took place at the hospital where the residents worked with patients in the psychiatry unit. Early in the lecture, Terry voiced a question he knew would be on the residents' minds: "Why even bother with [psychodynamic training]?" The answer, he asserted, lay with its distinctly valuable perspective: "The aim of having the psychodynamic psychotherapy experience, which is really not an insubstantial part of the residency here, is because there's really no other way to learn about patients' minds." Terry's assertion channeled long-simmering debates about the fate of psychiatry, pulled between "brainless" and "mindless" extremes.[1] His remarks did more than promise an expansion of the residents' professional repertoires. They also, if only implicitly, discredited their existing training. By focusing solely on symptoms and their management, Terry suggested, biological psychiatry would leave the residents unprepared to properly help their patients. Only a psychodynamic framework could help them care for patients and alleviate their suffering. But Terry knew that he could not simply teach the residents psychodynamic techniques. He also, and crucially, had to convince them of the value of learning a different way to doctor.

Shorewood instructors' manifest task was to broaden psychiatry residents' epistemic tool kits and teach them new ways to understand and treat mental illness. Yet the fundamental challenge they faced was making psychotherapy legitimate in a context that had rendered it not only secondary to biological treatments but also the domain of other mental health occupations. Terry's comments were typical of what instructors across orientations did to initiate the early psychiatrists into the world of psychotherapy. They stressed the advantages of doctoring psychotherapeutically and pointed to the shortcomings of biological approaches. They sought to establish the preeminence of their own therapeutic approach vis-à-vis various interventions, whether biological or talk and behavioral. They worked to make psychotherapeutic work legible to the residents' skeptical eyes.

In chapter 3, I showed the residents struggle with the loss of their epistemic and professional anchors as they began learning psychotherapy. In this chapter, I turn to psychotherapy instructors' own efforts to moor their trainees to new epistemic cultures. Psychotherapy instructors are more than passive targets of residents' doubts. They are, rather, key agents of the friction the residents experience and their principal interlocutors as they learn to navigate it. Much of the instructors' work is thus motivated by an awareness of the mismatches between doctoring therapeutically and doctoring pharmacologically, and by the need to naturalize and legitimize the former. Even as they know that the residents would not, by and large, go on to practice psychotherapy after graduation, the instructors are nevertheless invested in shifting the early psychiatrists' perspectives on the value and usefulness of talk and behavioral interventions.

The chapter begins with a discussion of Shorewood instructors' practical and discursive strategies for making psychotherapeutic expertise visible and, as such, believable. I show them conducting live sessions with patients and working to make their own tacit knowledge explicit through conversations about clinical cases. Together, these activities are central to instructors' efforts at opening up psychotherapeutic expertise for observation and apprenticing the residents into their craft. But the instructors also sought to make psychotherapeutic interventions legitimate to their skeptical audience by routinely engaging in what social scientists have described as symbolic boundary drawing, and I elaborate their approaches in the latter part of the chapter.[2] Their strategies of persuasion were aimed at distinguishing and extolling their own interventions as compared with other treatments for mental illness, be they pharmacological or talk therapeutic.

Making Therapeutic Expertise Visible

Apprenticeship depends on making experts' embodied knowledge visible such that novices can observe, emulate, and begin to internalize it.[3] Aware of the practical challenges the residents faced when confronted with doctoring without drugs, Shorewood instructors created opportunities for direct observation. With willing patients, they either conducted live sessions, typically behind one-way mirrors, or video recorded sessions to show at a later time. But the instructors also knew that such direct observation was insufficient for teaching residents what it means to think and feel psychotherapeutically. To foster this deeper know-how, they explained their approaches, revealing the thoughts and feelings that motivated their actions in session and offering the residents a backstage view of therapeutic expertise. In seeking to articulate their tacit knowledge, the experienced clinicians hoped to render psychotherapy comprehensible to the residents' novice eyes.

EXPERT THERAPISTS IN ACTION

The work of psychotherapy takes place behind closed doors, in conditions that sociologist Rose Laub Coser has described as "insulation from observability."[4] The arrangement is not unique to psychotherapy—indeed, much expert work is conducted in contexts manifestly set up to protect clients' privacy while also signaling the autonomy and authority of the professionals doing it.[5] Yet psychotherapists' commitment to privacy, a commitment that has taken its most acute form in psychodynamic approaches, has been particularly steadfast and has made training especially challenging. "We were thrown into this new situation," Jake, a graduating PGY-4, told Terry and Patricia during an end-of-year meeting of the psychodynamic group, "and we're all struggling logistically how to make it work!" The "new situation" Jake was invoking was doing psychodynamic psychotherapy during the second postgraduate year. He was careful to point out that the residents "all valued" the experience of learning the psychodynamic approach. But, he continued, "we were sitting there, like, 'OK, so what do we actually do?' You know?! Like, teach us the procedure if you will." These concerns, especially acute in psychodynamic psychotherapy, extended to cognitive behavioral therapy (CBT), where the residents wondered how to transition from talking with patients about their symptoms to talking about their thought patterns, or how to implement a particular technique or tool. During medical school and the beginning of residency, they had learned how to doctor by working alongside more experienced colleagues and attending psychiatrists, observing them talk with patients, make decisions about their care, and follow up on the effects of treatment. The residents had yet to see psychotherapy in action. Their instructors would help rectify this.

Direct Observation in Cognitive Behavioral Therapy

CBT skewed closer to the residents' biopsychiatric doctoring approach, but in observing their instructors actually put it into practice, they would find that here, too, they still had much to learn. Early in the CBT for depression rotation, Aaron (PGY-3), Turner (PGY-3), Sanjay (PGY-3), Jason (PGY-4), and I had the opportunity to see Robert, the experienced psychologist who trained the residents in this orientation, conduct an initial session with a patient, Rose. This was one of four such live demonstrations I would observe alongside residents in the CBT rotations.[6] Rose had come to the clinic seeking help with ongoing depression. She was already seeing Lucas (PGY-4) for medication management but wanted to taper off psychiatric drugs. Lucas had recommended CBT, and Rose had agreed to an initial session with Robert in a room outfitted with a one-way mirror. A few minutes before the session, the residents and I sat in the observation room while Robert handed out an "agenda," a list of tasks he set out to accomplish during this session. The agenda would help us follow along. It also served a practical purpose for the residents: it broke the process of doctoring in CBT into circumscribed tasks, offering a guide for how to navigate the forty-five-minute therapy session.

Robert started the meeting with Rose by assessing her symptoms and getting a better sense of the treatments she was undergoing at the time. For the residents, this was familiar terrain, a typical part of a psychiatric interview. But soon after, Robert began doing the kind of relational work with which the residents had less experience:

> *Robert (Instructor/Therapist)*: What I'd like to do today is catch up on how you've been doing and talk about how you feel about starting CBT here, and what you know about CBT and what you would like to work on. Does that sound like something that you would've expected to have happen today?
> *Rose (Patient)*: I'm not really familiar with what CBT is. . . . I just know that it's a form of talk therapy.

The residents and I had repeatedly heard CBT instructors stress the importance of "collaborating" with patients. Robert demonstrated just what that would mean, starting early in the session: he did not simply tell Rose what they would do during their time together but also asked her what she had "expected to have happen." Later, when she explained that "this particular brand of therapy" was unfamiliar to her, Robert validated her position: "Sure, so you'll know whether this can do something for you. Makes sense to me. That's one of the goals that I have today, to explain to you how it works and see if it makes sense to you."

Robert went on to explain the CBT model (one of the items on his agenda), telling Rose that "there's situations that happen to us in our lives and that in reaction to them we have thoughts, and in reaction to these thought patterns we have emotions. They are all connected, and we found that [by] targeting the thoughts, we can maybe change the emotions and the behaviors." But Rose was skeptical. She did not think that her "deeply ingrained" thoughts could be changed at all. Robert did not avoid nor delay addressing her disbelief. Instead, he moved to demonstrate how the model worked, asking: "Can you give me an example of a thought pattern that is really deeply ingrained? Or is that too much too soon?" Robert presaged his patient's reticence and reinforced the collaborative tone of the session, strengthening their incipient alliance. Rose went along, recalling a situation in which she did not join her coworkers on a social outing. Robert continued Rose's CBT education by explaining the difference between "preferences" that she would have "regardless of whether you are depressed or not" and those that are largely motivated by her depression. The former, Robert clarified, would not be a target of intervention in the treatment; it was the latter they would focus on in their work. Explicitly, he clarified that treatment would take up her depression and its manifestations. Implicitly, Robert also assured his skeptical patient that CBT would not seek to transform her very self.

At Robert's encouragement, Rose followed up with another, seemingly more ingrained belief:

Rose (Patient): I would say that I'm not the best mom in the world . . .

Robert (Instructor/Therapist): So on a scale of 0 to 10, how do you think [your children] would rate you as a parent?

[*Rose guesses that they would likely put her somewhere "in the middle."*]

Robert: And you would tend to agree with that assessment? [Rose nods.] So if you see that assessment, what kind of emotion does that trigger if you think about it?

Rose: Guilt . . .

Robert: And does that guilt at times get intense if you think about it?

[*Rose speaks briefly about times in her life when she felt guiltier than at present, as her relationships with her children had improved over time.*]

Robert: So it sounds like what might be most accurate is that your mothering ability varied over time. So again, from my cognitive and behavioral point of view, I would ask whether it's accurate to say that your mothering varied over time, and if it did, we would look at your guilt and what other kinds of thinking you could have about not being such a good parent some of the time. Is there any thinking that's going on there that might not be 100 percent reasonable? And we could try to change that. Does that make sense?

Robert knew that he could not move faster than his patient. But he was eager to quiet some of Rose's doubts about whether CBT could be useful to her. He thus did what I would come to recognize as a thought record exercise, without the actual form: he examined Rose's belief about her mothering (an unrealistic thought) by asking her to associate it with a feeling and to reflect on whether it was "100 percent reasonable." Then, as she identified fluctuations in the quality of her mothering, Robert could attempt to change her "deeply held" belief that she was not a good mother. After that quick demonstration of how CBT worked, Robert spent the rest of the session identifying the goals Rose wished to pursue in their work together. As the session neared its end, he recommended that she read the first three chapters of David Burns's book *Feeling Good*, that she schedule "ten sessions so we can have a time frame to work with," and that they meet once a week.[7]

Robert accomplished all the goals on the agenda: he helped "delineate [the patient's] specific problems," "establish treatment goals," and "talk about what CBT involves." He "elicit[ed the] patient's reactions to [the] CBT model" and her "prior expectations of therapy." He also did two cognitive exercises demonstrating the utility of the approach. Yet much of what Robert did was not on the handout he had shared with the residents. I was struck by his ability to seamlessly move between agenda items without rushing the patient along. He was attentive to Rose's doubts, acknowledging them but also seeking to undo them early on. For the residents, the session was a chance to see how they might doctor in CBT by bringing together the focus and concreteness they had come to expect in biopsychiatry with the relational and affective skills required in psychotherapy.

Direct Observation in Psychodynamic Psychotherapy

Psychodynamic psychotherapy was altogether more mysterious, as Jake's comments made clear. Here, direct observation could go a long way toward demystifying the approach. My initial observations at Shorewood took place when Terry conducted three "intake interviews" with Rob, a patient who had come to the clinic suffering from depression. This was also the residents' first opportunity to see psychodynamic psychotherapy in action. Prior to Terry's first session with Rob, the conference room where the psychodynamic group met was full of residents engaged in lively conversation. On a large screen, a video feed of Terry's session revealed a small windowless room furnished solely with two office chairs and a conference table. Terry moved the table to the side—his attempt at creating a space for intimacy and connection. Though at that point I had yet to visit the nearly sixty psychotherapy offices I would sit in during my fieldwork, I could already see why he would think the room was "austere," as he later described it. Video cameras added awkwardness for both patient and therapist (both had agreed to the recordings).

Over their three meetings together, Rob shared a rich personal history that included a tense relationship with his mother, several troubling mental health treatments, and a search for perfection. Even to my untrained eye it seemed that all this could make for a lengthy psychotherapy. The patient was conscious of his effect, commenting to Terry at the end of their first meeting: "How do you think the residents will like that?" The residents were indeed enthralled by Rob's story. They kept an ongoing hushed commentary about his disclosures—sometimes interrupted by laughter or gasps. Once, they tried to outdo one another guessing the medications Rob had been prescribed during an earlier hospitalization. Other times they commented on Rob's inability to express his emotions and questioned whether he withheld parts of his past. They were outsiders looking in, pharmacologists trying to make sense of a patient psychodynamically.

Terry's goal in conducting the interviews was to model a way of doctoring that diverged from the residents' own. He started the first session with an open-ended invitation to Rob: "Tell me about being depressed." As the patient recounted his academic and relationship troubles, Terry followed his lead, asking probing questions from time to time. When Rob described a passion for comic books as a way to "distract himself," Terry asked him, "What do you think you were trying to distract yourself from?" Inquiries such as "What was that like for you?" or "What did you make of that?" or, more pointedly, "What was going on inside your soul?" were crafted to encourage the patient to share more of his inner life.

Like other psychoanalytic clinicians I spoke with, Terry eschewed the use of a diagnostic inventory and did not conduct a typical psychiatric interview. Although diagnostic questions did appear, they were so minimally attended to and deftly woven into the conversation that it was not until I revisited my field notes that I came to recognize them as such. Instead, Terry focused on learning about Rob's "mind," to paraphrase his opening statement to the PGY-2s. He sought to get to know the patient "as a person." Doing so required Terry to attend less to Rob's medical history and more to his emotional and relational life. When Rob discussed a particularly stressful trip he had taken, Terry amplified his feelings: "Sounds like it was terrifying for you!" And when he apologized for having a "complicated" history, Terry reassured him: "It is complicated, but you don't have to be sorry! I mean, I'm sorry that you had to go through all that!" The experienced therapist focused on forming an empathetic relationship with the patient.

Terry modeled for the residents the basics of psychodynamic therapy: getting to know the patient beyond his diagnosis, creating a connection with him, and fostering introspection. He also showcased an essential psychodynamic technique: using his emotions to better understand the patient's. During his third session with Rob, the conversation in the therapy room turned, again, to the patient's early psychiatric hospitalization. When Terry asked how he felt about it, Rob put up a barrier, explaining that he had had to "repress" his feelings to be able to "go on with his life." Terry then tried an alternate tactic:

> *Terry (Instructor/Therapist):* Let me ask you about something: as we're talking about it, it appears to me that I'm getting more upset about this than you are! What do you make of that difference? As you're talking about it, it seems like you're saying that you didn't have such a great lunch [. . .]!
> *Rob (Patient)* [*Responds that he does not want to "let [himself] feel."*]
> *Terry:* Why not? What is it that kept you from letting yourself feel? Somehow, if you let yourself feel, you would not have been able to have a relationship with your parents [who were responsible for the hospitalization]? I still don't know what [your doctors] were medicating you for. That's how [your doctors and your parents] thought you felt, but how did *you* feel?

Seeking to better understand Rob, Terry made a direct appeal to his own reactions. The exchange showcased the workings of what psychoanalysts call *countertransference*—attending to their own feelings as significant data about the interaction and, sometimes, about patients themselves. But Rob was determined to hold back. For Terry, this reticence only provided another entry point: "Why" didn't Rob want to "let [himself] feel"? He put into practice the very techniques I would see him repeatedly offer residents frustrated by their own patients' inability or unwillingness to disclose.

The residents were learning how to be with patients without the use of symptom checklists and prescription pens. Through the video feed, they saw Terry get to know Rob intimately by asking him questions not just about his illness but about his life. They also observed Terry use humor and irony to create a connection with Rob. When the patient revealed that he has dozens of cousins on his father's side, Terry remarked, "That's a heck of a barbecue!" On another occasion, at the end of their three sessions together, during a discussion about what would work best for Rob's treatment moving forward, Terry asked:

> *Terry (Instructor/Therapist):* Do you have a sense for the kind of person that would be most helpful to you? How do you feel about the idea of working with somebody else after this?
> *Rob (Patient)* [*hesitantly*]: Well, you seem good.
> *Terry* [*in a half-serious tone*]: Well, at least we know your reality check is correct!

I laughed along with the residents at Terry's jokes. As the laughter died down after this exchange, Patricia pointed out that Terry was "using humor" to "soften the blow" of having to end the nascent relationship he had built with Rob. Terry's levity complemented his easy but engaged and attentive manner. Rob seemed to respond to it well, evidenced by his desire to continue treatment together. Terry had deployed the right mix of curiosity, warmth, empathy, humor, and expertise. As he displayed his own approach to doctoring, the residents saw that they need not maintain an impenetrable facade of "clinical empathy" in their relationships with patients.[8] When one resident laughingly remarked that Terry "says some awful shit sometimes!" in response to the psychoanalyst's barbecue quip, another, also laughing, pointed out, "It works, though!" This was the collective management of skepticism in action.

DEMONSTRATING TACIT KNOWLEDGE

From behind the one-way mirror or the video screen, the residents could learn how to do therapy by watching experienced clinicians with patients. They observed their instructors conduct sessions, introduce patients to the treatment approach, and ask about their troubles. They heard them frame patients' problems in therapy-specific terms, balance directiveness with restraint, and lay the groundwork for therapeutic relationships. Yet even as such direct observations were useful, they did not reveal the knowledge their instructors drew on in their work. All the residents could see was what Robert and Terry did and said in the therapy room. But they did not have access to the thought processes that motivated the experienced clinicians' actions and words.[9] As Turner (PGY-3) remarked during the discussion that followed Robert's session with Rose, a "big part of the session was not on this [agenda] sheet." Neither the agenda nor the accompanying observation could tell the residents everything they needed to know about doctoring therapeutically, partly because the instructors were experts with stores of what social scientists have called "tacit knowledge."[10] Tacit knowledge is tethered to practice and difficult to articulate. It is a marker of expertise, stemming from prolonged immersion in an epistemic culture, its norms, rituals, and practices. The instructors had had years to hone their therapeutic know-how, bringing to sessions not only their knowledge of psychoanalytic or cognitive behavioral theories and techniques but also the embodied skills of talking with and relating to patients. They sought to make such knowledge visible to the residents through discussions following each session. Whether they pointed out when they "had to repress a smile," as Terry did with Rob, or performed the "Columbo approach," as Jeremy, the CBT for anxiety instructor described it—that is, not trying to "match wits" with his patient and instead talking "very slowly without using big words," as exemplified by Peter Falk's classic TV police detective—such conversations were meant to make psychotherapeutic expertise visible.

This happened typically during debriefings that followed live sessions. Often, these conversations revealed the disjunctures the residents perceived between biopsychiatric doctoring and the psychotherapeutic models they saw their instructors inhabit. After Robert's session with Rose, the residents and I returned to the conference room for a brief discussion of what we had witnessed. Aaron (PGY-3) was especially interested in Robert's choices about when to intervene and when to listen. Though I had been struck by how quickly Robert had moved to implementing CBT interventions, Aaron remarked on his patience:[11]

> *Aaron (PGY-3)*: I think I tend to jump ahead, and I was kind of surprised that you were sitting back and talking about the goals [of treatment]. . . . You were just kind of observing and taking it in, and I would hear guilt and I would want to jump on it as a cognitive distortion, and that comes later and it's not something you want to do right away.
> [. . .]
> *Robert (Instructor)*: What would be the risk of doing that?
> *Aaron*: You probably would scare them away, you kind of risk alienating the patient . . .
> *Robert*: Particularly for a patient that she describes being shy and the importance to feel safe, I would want it to unfold a little more slowly. [. . .] It's easy for the person to feel like they're being criticized or that you're telling them how to think, and they can get defensive.

Aaron was used to identifying a problem and moving quickly to a (pharmacological) solution. This had been the pace of his work at the hospital, and it remained his dominant approach during medication management appointments at the clinic. In CBT, he would learn not only an alternate means to work with patients but also the drawbacks of his existing technique when misapplied. Making a patient "feel like they're being criticized" would be easy in a treatment focused on identifying "distorted" or "unrealistic" thoughts. Whereas some patients may be more amenable to moving faster toward change, Rose, Robert noted, was "shy" and needed to "feel safe." Robert explained: "I made a note to myself to try to build the relationship, so you noticed that I was paraphrasing what she said for the purpose of making her feel safe and build the relationship." A slower pace that strengthened the relationship and fostered trust would be more appropriate for this particular patient. As Robert elaborated on his thinking, he helped the residents understand some of the tacit work he performed to ensure the success of the session and lay a foundation for what could be a difficult treatment.

Robert's session with Rose made expert therapeutic work look seamless. The discussion revealed the less visible cognitive and affective effort that Robert had expended to pull it off. Deploying the right words at the right time and attending to the patient's doubts as much as to the treatment's progression were just some of the challenges that the experienced psychotherapist could navigate with ease. By making his tacit knowledge visible to the residents, Robert made clear that even in CBT—where they could rely on agendas, forms, and exercises—doctoring required more than learning rules and techniques. Instead, it necessitated a constant tuning between therapist and patient and depended on therapists' awareness of themselves as much as of their patients.

In psychodynamic training, the residents' questions for Terry reflected their ongoing concerns with how they might make sense of patients' problems if symptoms and diagnoses were not useful, and how they might gain access to their inner lives without the use of questionnaires and directive interviewing. The conversation that followed Terry's first session with Rob turned to the patient's "chief complaint." Was it his depression? His inability to complete his graduate work? A "chief complaint" would, in addition to Rob's symptoms, inform treatment, at least in the residents' pharmacological playbook. But Terry wanted to shift the residents' attention away from these considerations. He explained that he had employed a different "diagnostic strategy" during the session. "At one point I said, 'I'm confused.' There are a number of ways in which a patient can respond to that," Terry continued. He could say, "What the fuck is wrong with you?" or "I can understand your being confused, so let me go back and explain." These disparate answers, Terry explained, would reveal something about the patient's ability to relate to others. "[Rob] did the latter," Terry pointed out, "which means that he can make an alliance and empathize," key indicators of an ability to engage in psychodynamic treatment. Terry did more than share with the residents a practical strategy (telling the patient that he was "confused"). He also explained why he employed it and how he interpreted the patient's response. This is the kind of knowledge-in-action that would have gone unnoticed by the residents, focused as they were on the patient's "chief complaint."

A conversation after a different session revealed how Terry approached another arena that proved challenging for the residents: learning about patients' emotions. The residents were troubled by the patient's aversion or, possibly, inability to discuss his feelings. Zaheed (PGY-3) noticed that Terry had "named some [of Rob's] feelings" during session. Searching for a guiding principle, Zaheed asked, "Do you usually do that with patients, or do you let them describe their feelings?" Terry explained that Rob "was not replete with adjectives," putting the therapist in a position of having to "name" some of the patient's feelings. "But," he cautioned, "therapists have to be careful with patients because some can be very suggestible, so you must be careful when you name the feelings, versus when you ask the patient to describe them themselves." The residents did not yet benefit from the kind of accumulated experience that Terry could draw on to know when to pose particular kinds of questions and how they might affect patients. What the experienced analyst could offer was a conceptually simple but practically challenging rule: "follow the affect"—their patients' and their own—to figure out what works.

Jarvis (PGY-4), a more experienced resident, remarked on a moment during the first session when Terry did comment on one of Rob's expressions of emotion: "You actually said something when he laughed at his mention of 9/11; you said, 'You're laughing *now!*'"[12] Jarvis had noticed Terry's efforts at drawing out Rob's emotional life and implicitly invited him to explain his strategy. Terry clarified: "I find it helpful to let someone know that I am noticing their affect." This was a basic therapeutic lesson about demonstrating empathy. But, Terry continued, his thinking went deeper than simple empathy: "This guy was creating 9/11s wherever he goes." Nevertheless, even as he became embroiled in emotionally volatile situations, the patient, Terry explained, had "spent the last fifteen years of his life pushing stuff down." Terry was drawing the residents' attention to the unconscious dynamics he was beginning to think about. He was also making clear that his interactions with Rob were driven both by moment-to-moment judgments about empathy and relatedness and by larger concerns with putting together a story about the patient's life.

These discussions, along with opportunities to observe psychotherapy instructors with patients, offered the residents valuable entry points into psychotherapy. That they were also avenues for the management of skepticism became abundantly clear when the residents watched recorded psychotherapy sessions that showed renowned practitioners—typically in CBT—at work. In conversations with their Shorewood instructors, the residents' doubts were at times obscured by displays of novice uncertainty. But after watching recordings of Albert Ellis, Judith Beck, and other experienced CBT clinicians—clinicians with whom the residents did not have any direct contact nor long-term relationships—the residents freely expressed their skepticism and critiques.[13] Whether a therapist was "doing all [the] work for" his patient rather than enabling her to do it herself, or gave her patient "too much" to do and "was all over the place," the clinicians in the videos were found wanting. Patients, the residents thought, would feel "overwhelmed" by the sessions or, alternatively, find the approach "too simple" or commonsense. Seeing their own instructors in action was thus about more than exposure to the practice of therapy. It was also about legitimizing psychotherapeutic interventions and expertise.

Making Therapeutic Expertise Legitimate

Psychotherapy instructors were conscious of the barriers they had to surmount when training psychiatry residents. They knew that they could not simply focus on imparting practical knowledge about their approaches to these skeptical novices. After all, they, too, had experienced some of the same epistemic and professional friction when they had to coordinate several kinds of care for their patients.[14] Instructors thus aimed to allay the residents' doubts by appealing both to their knowledge of the field and to their clinical experience. They engaged in what social scientists have called *symbolic boundary work*, the process of drawing "conceptual distinctions" in negotiations of status, power, and belonging.[15] Members of distinct social groups use cultural resources and practices—such as forms of aesthetic expression, consumption, stories and narratives, or traditions and rituals—to set themselves apart from each other. In the world of professions, symbolic boundary work revolves around claims making—about evidence, facts, objectivity, commitments—by which groups shore up their power.[16] For psychotherapy instructors, boundary work was thus a means to establish the legitimacy of their own approach to an audience socialized to treat psychotherapy as secondary to biological psychiatry.

INSTRUCTORS COMPARING PSYCHOTHERAPY FAVORABLY TO BIOPSYCHIATRY

"Some of the articles that you referred us recently on the neuroscience and psychodynamic intersection have been helpful in conceptualizing how development plays into the brain," Vinit, a PGY-4 who was weeks away from graduation, told Terry and Patricia during an end-of-year group conversation.[17] "'Cause it's almost like, we almost need to be sold on this being a legitimate [intervention]." Undoubtedly because of his impending graduation, Vinit was surprisingly honest. Early in their training, he explained, the residents heard "a lot of misinformation [. . .] that influences our perspective [on psychodynamic psychotherapy], so being sold on it, it's like huge! It's a hurdle to go over before we start learning!" Terry was in the habit of invoking neuroscientific research as a way of confirming long-accepted psychoanalytic theories. The articles and references, it turned out, were not only useful for elucidating scientific questions or psychoanalytic concepts. As Vinit made clear, they were also "really, really helpful" in mitigating some of the residents' skepticism.

Felix, another PGY-4 nearing graduation, echoed Vinit's perspective: "We do the first two years in a highly biologically oriented environment." There, he clarified, "some people have a lot of respect for the psychodynamically oriented approach, and [encourage] us to learn it. Other people don't, and have the opposite stance."[18] Terry took this as an opportunity to blur the boundaries between biopsychiatry and psychodynamics that Felix and his colleagues had internalized earlier in their training: "It's funny, because I think that in fact what we do is a biological approach. It's a different set of techniques, but it's not any less biological than other approaches!" To support his assertion, Terry referenced the work of historian of science Frank Sulloway, whose biography of Sigmund Freud argued that, in Terry's telling, the founder of psychoanalysis "was operating from a very biologically based paradigm and it tainted all of his work."[19] Though one might quibble with the proposition that Freud's biological interests and research would have shaped a field that has been developing over more than a hundred years across multiple continents,[20] Terry's message to the residents was clear: psychodynamic psychotherapy and biological psychiatry had a shared history that revolved around understanding the relationship between mind and brain.

Jeremy, the psychologist who ran the CBT for anxiety rotation, identified a different zone of affinity between psychotherapy and biological psychiatry, and between mental health and the larger field of medicine. "Our patients have the expectation that our treatments are curative," he explained to his trainees. "And if they didn't cure you for the rest of your life, then it's a failure and it's time for a different approach." Yet patients are mistaken, Jeremy asserted: "Our treatments here in psychiatry are just like any others. The mental problem may come back. Nowhere else in the field of health care can we expect that a problem is solved forever." Jeremy's comments hinted at the common terrain that psychotherapy and biological psychiatry inhabited. By using the adverb "our" and contrasting "psychiatry" with the rest of medicine, Jeremy suggested that psychotherapy and pharmacology shared more common ground with each other than one might assume.

Whether they sought to highlight the convergence between biological psychiatry and psychotherapy by pointing out their common commitments or their limitations, Terry and Jeremy were blurring the symbolic boundaries dividing them. All the while, they were participating in the management of skepticism necessary for cooperating in spaces where distinct epistemic cultures meet. Yet pointing to such overlaps was only one strategy for doing so. Though telling, their efforts at reconciling psychotherapy and biological psychiatry were nevertheless rare. More frequently, they and other instructors sought to establish their own approach's superiority to biological treatments. In an environment where medications seemed to be the solution to every mental illness problem, the instructors' efforts reminded residents that there are useful and legitimate nonchemical alternatives.

Whether they admonished the residents about the importance of learning about patients' minds, as Terry put it in his comments to the PGY-2s, or offered them concrete strategies for helping those who did not get better with medications, instructors took every opportunity to stress the advantages of talk and behavioral interventions. Frequently, they appealed to their clinical experience to extol psychotherapy's successes. On countless occasions I heard instructors answer the residents' questions and meet their doubts about a therapeutic assumption or technique by talking about a patient they had treated successfully with that very approach.

Such strategies were even more compelling when they referred to patients with whom the residents were already familiar. This was the case with Meredith, a patient suffering from obsessive-compulsive disorder (OCD) who was being treated at the clinic by Luna, an experienced CBT therapist. Luna was an expert in anxiety disorders, OCD in particular, and she helped train novices in this approach. On one occasion, Luna asked Meredith whether she would agree to a session in front of the CBT training group consisting of three residents, two social workers, one psychologist, and me. Meredith agreed. Before the session started, Luna asked her patient to share her previous treatment experiences with us. Meredith, a married mother of two with perfectly applied makeup and coiffed hair, recounted seeing "a few counselors and therapists" and undergoing three hospitalizations. But "nobody knew specifically what to do." As her illness got worse and her life began to fall apart, Meredith decided to make the nearly two-hour drive to see someone at Shorewood. "Coming here and meeting with [Luna]," Meredith explained, "I could tell right away that she knew what to do with the OCD." "Nobody has known what to do," Meredith stressed, but Luna had been the exception.

As Meredith explained what she had found helpful about the treatment— Luna's description of the interplay between thoughts and emotions in OCD, her gradual approach, the treatment strategies—she painted a convincing picture of her progress. Luna's method had made sense to Meredith. Significantly, it had already started to show results, as Meredith was becoming "desensitized" to the emotional effects of her repetitive thoughts and was regaining her "confidence" in her ability to face the illness. Meredith's words alone made for compelling testimony. The difficult work she undertook during the session, made harder by emotions that ranged from hesitance to sobbing, made clear that what she offered was not empty praise.

But it was Luna's comments after the session that really stood out to me. After everyone had thanked Meredith for her time and willingness to work on her problems in a room full of trainees, and she left, Luna turned to the group and explained:

> One of the main reasons I wanted [Meredith] to be here today is to give you guys an idea of how frustrated and how angry it makes me that exposure has been around, and it's been an evidence-based treatment for twenty-five years, and that this woman had two experiences in the hospital and three years of therapy before somebody said, "You have OCD, [and] you need to go see someone who does exposure!" And I think that very often what happens with these intrusive violent thoughts is that people are scared of them. And they shy away from doing what needs to be done because it makes them feel uncomfortable!

Luna's choice of adjectives and stern tone made clear the urgency she felt in teaching the residents and their colleagues exposure therapy. "Psychiatry," Luna stressed, had not "not done a whole lot for" Meredith. The patient had suffered through several years of unsuccessful treatments, each leaving her more troubled and discouraged. Luna positioned the residents and other trainees as witnesses to the limitations and even harms that result from improper treatments begotten by psychiatry's commitment to biology. By learning how to conduct "exposure" interventions, the residents would be better equipped to avoid such failures.

In psychodynamic psychotherapy, Terry and Patricia also made impassioned appeals in favor of their approach. One such instance stood out for the stark distinction Terry painted between biological psychiatry and psychodynamic psychotherapy. During another end-of-year discussion, this time with the PGY-3s, the instructors had listened as the residents spent the better part of an hour describing their difficulties transitioning from working with hospitalized patients to doing psychodynamic psychotherapy. Toward the end of the hour Terry wanted to establish, again, the value of psychodynamic training. "Fundamentally, our first responsibility is to know our patients," he stressed. "Human beings are amazing, exquisite beings, and to not have that, from my perspective, is tragic." Psychiatrists are not "computer programmers," Terry asserted. "If you come out of this experience with nothing else other than the attitude that people are incredibly interesting, [then] we will have met that priority." Psychiatry had failed to cultivate the residents' appreciation of their patients' humanity. Only in psychodynamic psychotherapy could they develop this more generous and compassionate perspective. Seeing Terry work with Rob, and hearing the patient express a desire to continue treatment with the experienced analyst, made for compelling testimony to the perspective's utility.

INSTRUCTORS EXTOL THEIR OWN
PSYCHOTHERAPEUTIC APPROACH

In a field where treatment effectiveness continues to be debated, the boundaries that need management are not simply those between psychotherapy and biological psychiatry but also those within psychotherapy proper.[21] The experienced clinicians I observed were thus not simply concerned with showing the residents that psychotherapy was as helpful or even, at times, more helpful than psychiatric drugs. They also, just as frequently, set their sights on other psychotherapeutic approaches. Despite momentary attention to areas of overlap, senior therapists, along with the dozens of other clinicians I spoke with as part of this research, talked freely about what they viewed as the fault lines between cognitive behavioral treatments (e.g., CBT, dialectical behavioral therapy [DBT]), interpersonal psychotherapy (IPT), and psychodynamic psychotherapy. Practitioners of CBT, DBT, or IPT described their interventions as "evidence-based" or "empirically supported," "effective," "efficient," and "goal oriented." For their part, psychodynamic therapists and psychoanalysts stressed that their own methods attended to the "whole person," providing patients with a path toward lasting change rather than temporary symptom relief.

The residents were prime audiences for such contestations. When one resident asked how they might decide which psychotherapeutic treatment would be most appropriate for a patient, Robert, the CBT for depression instructor, asserted:

> In terms of CBT and DBT versus psychodynamic, I always think [CBT and DBT are] better because they're empirically supported. . . . In terms of the people who would be better for [psycho]dynamic are those who really want it, who say they have things in their past that they want to sort out, or they want to do longer-term therapy. . . . But for those people who feel more distressed and need to do something about it quickly, then I always recommend CBT and DBT.

Though patients' preferences mattered, Robert made clear that CBT and its offshoot, DBT, were "better." He turned to a common justification to bolster his point: these approaches were "empirically supported"; they had the weight of scientific evidence on their side and offered patients faster relief. Psychodynamic therapy was for those who suffered less acutely and were more interested in "sorting out" "things in their past." While not outright dismissing CBT's competitor, Robert made plain that there was only one set of interventions that actually helped patients in "distress."

Psychodynamic instructors were similarly keen to impress on the residents the utility of their own approach. During a conversation in the psychodynamic psychotherapy rotation about the importance of the psychotherapeutic relationship, Terry remarked:

> I think [. . .] the reason that people go into psychodynamic therapy is different than going into CBT and IPT [interpersonal therapy]. And that is that they don't understand what's going on in their relationships, and we are there to help them understand that. . . . And that in some ways is out of the bounds of those other [treatment] relationships. [Our work] is absolutely unique and it doesn't happen in any other kind of therapy.

Psychodynamic psychotherapy's "unique" contribution was to help patients understand the troubles afflicting their relationships. For Terry and other psychoanalytically inclined clinicians, it was the only way to understand what caused patients' suffering and help them overcome it. Symptoms would get resolved as patients deepened their knowledge of themselves, came to recognize their relational patterns, and began to change them. None of this work, Terry made clear, was possible in other therapeutic frameworks.

Psychotherapy instructors offered the residents distinct visions of what was best for patients, each convinced of the advantages of their own approach. Even Robert's concession that there are some "people who would be better for [psycho]dynamic" can be viewed as an implicit rebuttal of the approach: sorting out "things in their past" is not the same as treating patients who are "distressed." Such comments should not be taken as simply talk. The residents were simultaneously learning multiple psychotherapeutic modalities, and their instructors were frequently confronted with the task of having to disentangle their thinking and explain the value of their own intervention.

Instructors' work of distinction was especially important early in the residents' psychotherapy training when their budding knowledge disposed them to recognize commonalities rather than differences between approaches. Then, too, instructors could intervene to distinguish their preferred method. Two months into my fieldwork, the residents' tendency to integrate therapeutic approaches became evident as one of the residents sought to link psychodynamic psychotherapy and behaviorism:

> *Draymond (PGY-3)*: Dr. S [Terry], so we're trying to basically help patients through exposure therapy?

> *Terry (Instructor)*: Yes, but we're exposing them to their own feelings. . . .
> Now, why do this in a dynamic rather than a behavioral way? Why not
> take the abused child and sit him down and just show him videos of
> other children being abused?
>
> *Leah (PGY-3)*: Because of the transference . . . because that child's experi-
> ence of his abuse was probably different from the ones that he would
> be seeing in the video. . . . Because many things can trigger a particular
> memory.
>
> *Terry*: An open-ended psychodynamic approach allows for most possibilities
> to be explored.

Terry did not reject outright Draymond's suggestion that there are
some similarities between psychodynamic and behavioral interventions.
One could describe psychodynamic therapy's goals as "exposing" patients
"to their own feelings," the analyst agreed, but this would understate its
potential. Patients would be best helped not by a reliance on behavioral
"exposure" treatments nor, for that matter, on pharmacological ones. The
residents needed instead to understand each patient's specific experiences.
Terry's caricature of the behavioral treatment ("take the abused child and
sit him down"), was intended to convince the residents that psychodynamic psychotherapy would be the better intervention because it would
attend to the patient's unique suffering and life course.

In the CBT for depression rotation, Turner (PGY-3) was similarly struck
by similarities between CBT and psychodynamic psychotherapy. His comment created an opening for Robert's own intervention:

> *Turner (PGY-3)*: I know that we've talked before in here about schemas, but
> I'm not entirely sure that I have an automatic grasp of that yet. [. . .]
> It makes me think that [CBT] is a lot like psychodynamic therapy, you
> know, the idea of talking about [the patient's] parents . . .
>
> *Robert (Instructor)*: That reaction often happens . . . It does illustrate that
> there's some similarity between cognitive therapy and psychodynamic
> therapy because we do look at how patients grew up and [try] to figure
> out how their thoughts and beliefs came about. But then we focus on
> the here and now, solving the problems of the present. I was doing this
> with a patient, and he can see that if he knows where those beliefs came
> from, they're not universal truths, and they can be undone. We don't
> dwell there.

Robert could not fully dismiss psychodynamic psychotherapy. After all,
cognitive therapy developed out of the fertile ground of psychoanalysis.[22]
Schemas, the concept that gave Turner pause, are deeply held beliefs about

the world that, Robert conceded, are rooted in "how patients grew up." But exploring such schemas, the experienced clinician stressed, was a means to an end, not an end in itself—as they would be, in Robert's telling, in psychodynamic psychotherapy. In CBT this could help patients understand that their beliefs are "not universal truths" and thus that they "can be undone." Such knowledge would then lay the groundwork for the real work of CBT: changing patients' thinking and "solving the problems of the present."

The focus and efficiency of shorter treatments were frequently held up as counterpoints to psychodynamic psychotherapy. During one initial meeting of the CBT rotation, Robert told the residents that, at the start of a treatment, he typically "suggests" to patients that they meet for "ten sessions"—and they saw him doing so with Rose, the patient whose treatment they observed from behind a one-way mirror. Aaron, an early PGY-3 and CBT novice, was taken aback: "Is it accepted to just set up a number of sessions?" "In CBT we set up some parameters that we will be working with," Robert affirmed, "rather than working indefinitely." The final adverb, "indefinitely," was a not-so-subtle reference to the psychodynamic model in which a treatment's length is, at least theoretically, open-ended. Such open-endedness was anathema to CBT. The image of an interminable psychodynamic treatment or psychoanalysis—not entirely baseless, but, as I would learn during my research, much less common than typically assumed—serves an important symbolic role in CBT.[23] It works as a tool for distinguishing CBT and related interventions from its epistemic predecessor, psychoanalysis. Unlike psychoanalysis and, by extension, psychodynamic psychotherapy, CBT is portrayed as efficient, effective, goal oriented, and financially feasible.

Instructors in this and other "empirically supported" interventions invoked common tropes to highlight these differences. Holly, the experienced psychologist who led the IPT rotation, alerted the residents: "Remember, this therapy doesn't work if changes aren't happening, if the person is not better and not making any changes. It's not insight-oriented therapy primarily, it's action-oriented therapy." I had heard numerous CBT practitioners contrast "insight" and "action." They described their approach as "active" because it required them and their patients to practice particular techniques and interventions. This was not a value-neutral description. It hinted at the purported capacities and efforts of therapists themselves. "Active" therapists, these clinicians implied, *worked* to get their patients better. They had concrete plans and skills to teach patients. Just as a medical doctor would give a patient a medication prescription, so a CBT clinician would send a patient home with exercises, homework they were to do on their own.

The residents reflected this language. When Sonora, a PGY-4 completing a fellowship in child psychiatry, told her reluctant patient Sam that "it's gonna take work" for him to get better, she did so to convey that he needed to complete his CBT "homework." This work "can be challenging," but, she assured him, his anxiety would lessen because of it. Two months into his treatment she had to reiterate that "this kind of therapy is [an] active therapy" that depended on Sam's engagement. The implicit contrast here was to a supportive or psychodynamic approach wherein the patient had to come to session and talk—seemingly Sam's preferred mode of care. The emphasis placed on change, work, and action served to distinguish CBT from the interventions of their psychodynamic colleagues.

Aware of this common narrative, psychodynamic clinicians in turn sought to reframe the implicit claim that their approach was "passive." In my conversations with therapists in this orientation, I heard them speak about the emotional and intellectual labor involved in facilitating patients' understanding, or "insight," as these therapists called it. Knowledge of one's patients—and patients' own subsequent knowledge of themselves—required effort and expertise. It also required patience, since—as I was frequently told—patients would arrive at such insight at their own pace. A therapist's silence, common in psychodynamic sessions, should thus not be taken for inaction. Ted, an experienced psychoanalyst who served as supervisor to some of the residents and sometimes came to talk to the group about an ongoing case, spoke of the importance of "staying in your chair" to reassure and support patients through their emotional work. Terry elaborated:

Ted described it beautifully, which is the myth of the passive therapist. I mean, [he] isn't saying very much, but he's doing a lot of work, and there's a lot of work that's implicit in [. . .] choosing to go down one path versus another and this isn't sort of the passive, unresponsive therapist, that is the stereotype of therapy! [That] is very wrong! He's just not talking a lot!

Ted had already discussed the difficulties he had overcome helping his patient talk about her feelings without rushing toward an understanding of what they might mean. Patricia pointed out that Ted's affective and verbal restraint had allowed the patient "to feel safe." Creating the feeling of "safety" and allowing the patient the freedom to talk about her life and her feelings without overwhelming her with interpretations was the analyst's active, though also mostly silent, work. The analyst was, in Terry's telling, a "coconspirator" with the patient, seeking to make inroads toward "understanding." This was not the "unresponsive therapist," a "stereotype" that psychodynamic clinicians fought against, but rather a therapist who is "just not talking a lot" yet still *working* to understand the patient. The "passive therapist" is a "myth" whose staying power psychodynamic instructors and supervisors were compelled to undo.

The experienced clinicians' perspectives were more than empty talk aimed at rhetorically establishing the worth of their own approach. They could in fact shape the residents' decisions about how to care for their patients. As doctors, residents could influence a patient's choice of treatment, including psychotherapy. When Sanjay (PGY-3) asked for Robert's advice about when it would be appropriate to "intrude" on a patient's psychodynamic treatment, the experienced CBT clinician urged, "You do want to tell the patient that there is evidence that [CBT and DBT] work for his kinds of problems." The patient would ultimately have to "make a decision about what he wants," but the resident's duty was to inform him "that it would be legitimate to get into a different form of therapy," especially if the resident, as his doctor, thought he "could benefit more from" another approach.

The residents found themselves in the crosshairs of such turf wars. Their positions as referral nodes meant that psychotherapy instructors' symbolic boundary drawing—extolling their own interventions and downplaying those of competitors—could be consequential for patients and mental health care providers alike. From a training perspective, disagreements among psychotherapy instructors about which intervention worked best could have dual consequences. On the one hand, by bringing to the foreground fissures in the field, such disagreements only added to the epistemic friction inherent in the residents' roles, heightening their skepticism toward psychotherapy training. On the other hand, instructors' boundary drawing opened spaces for the residents to craft their own paths toward competence. Faced with an unsettled field, the residents were not compelled to choose one intervention or another—they could, as I will show in chapter 7, develop distinct solutions to the problem of having to learn multiple, contrasting epistemic approaches.

Conclusion

The work of legitimation is not simply fought in professional journals and research programs. It is also an everyday preoccupation for clinicians who have to convince patients and colleagues alike about the value of their own interventions. Training programs are particularly fertile grounds for such symbolic work, particularly since they function as primary sites for shaping the epistemic and professional imaginaries of future practitioners. And while training psychiatrists in psychotherapy may seem inconsequential— after all, most residents go on to practice pharmacology after graduation— the stakes are significant. Psychiatrists' influence extends beyond patients' medication prescriptions to include referrals that shape what therapy they might receive and which practitioners would deliver it.

Shorewood instructors' work was thus doubly important. On the one hand, they had to equip the residents with the necessary epistemic tools to recognize when their patients needed something other than medications and to know how to help them. On the other hand, they had to render nonchemical treatments both viable and essential in a field that had marginalized them. Though their mandates were shaped by program and field-wide dynamics, putting them into practice placed psychotherapy instructors in the paradoxical position of being principal purveyors of the residents' friction and mediators of their skepticism. The instructors met these challenges by opening psychotherapeutic work and expertise to observation and by engaging in symbolic boundary work.

Their efforts at rendering therapeutic expertise observable were essential to the residents' apprenticeship in talk and behavioral approaches. As social scientists have shown, visibility facilitates the transmission of knowledge, particularly the tacit knowledge that is difficult to communicate didactically.[24] The residents' education in psychotherapy depended on being able to see expert therapists at work; they did so from behind one-way mirrors, through live video feeds, or even by being in the same room with therapists and their patients. Even as such live demonstrations happened infrequently, their efficaciousness was buttressed by group conversations in which experienced clinicians revealed the tacit knowledge that informed their decisions about patient care. Knowing what their instructors thought or felt in particular instances and how that influenced what they did with their patients in session helped the residents along the path of acquiring new doctoring repertoires.

More than apprenticeship, observation also facilitated legitimation. Visibility has the power to convince. Science and technology scholars have long shown that the credibility of scientific claims depends partly on their demonstrability. Opening scientific work to observation by what historian of science Steven Shapin has called the "witnessing public" renders it, and the claims makers themselves, credible.[25] To borrow Shapin's metaphor, psychotherapy instructors turned the residents into witnesses who could learn therapy *and* be convinced by what they saw. As they observed their instructors with patients, the residents witnessed their performances of expertise and patients' reactions. They could hear patients respond to the therapist's questions in ways that furthered the treatment and see them share more of their inner lives. They could sense the reverberations of empathy into the therapeutic relationship. At times, they could hear patients' doubts echo their own (will this therapy work?) and be met with instructors' justifications and encouragement.

Instructors' focus on legitimation extended beyond rendering psychotherapeutic expertise intelligible to the residents. The instructors also engaged in

symbolic boundary work, drawing favorable comparisons between psychotherapy and biopsychiatry, or between their own therapeutic approach and
alternative ones. Already cued to the affinities between CBT and biopsychiatry, the residents were primed to be more responsive to CBT instructors' work
of legitimation. In contrast, the psychodynamic team had a more challenging
path toward managing skepticism. For them, the stakes of the residents' acceptance of and competence in psychodynamic psychotherapy extended beyond this particular group or program. They reflected debates about the very
place of the psychodynamic approach in psychiatric education. I began my
fieldwork nearly a decade after the reinstatement of psychodynamic psychotherapy as a required area of proficiency for psychiatry trainees. Still, concerns regarding the evidentiary basis for psychodynamic approaches echoed
those of earlier decades, and skepticism toward its utility remained. In my
observations, such doubts made appearances in conversations between instructors and residents about the kind of treatment that may benefit a patient.
While CBT practitioners described their approaches as "evidence-based" or
"empirically supported"—thus making them legitimately medical—the psychoanalysts were put in a position to justify the utility of their approach as
well as, implicitly, the program's demands on the residents' time, by explaining the work that seemingly "passive" clinicians do.

For the residents, larger questions about observability and legitimacy
crystallized in the epistemic and professional friction in their roles and
the practical challenges of learning how to doctor psychotherapeutically.
While observing their instructors conduct sessions with patients was productive, it was nevertheless insufficient for building the residents' skills
and confidence in psychotherapy. Willingly or not, the residents had to
inhabit roles as therapy novices. Though treating patients was a crucial
component of training, the instructors knew well that, aside from psychodynamic psychotherapy, the residents were not always able or even willing
to take on psychotherapy patients—a refusal that functioned as one of the
few avenues for them to exercise a modicum of control.

In this context, the weekly meetings the residents attended as part of
the psychotherapy rotations were quite significant. Here, the psychiatrists could learn psychotherapy by presenting clinical cases and discussing
their own and their colleagues' treatment conundrums. Group meetings
were particularly propitious contexts in which the residents could begin
to try out therapeutic roles. And they could do so in the company of their
colleagues who were facing similar struggles and would thus make for a
generous audience. The next two chapters detail these processes and the
residents' own experiences, illuminating their struggles learning to doctor psychotherapeutically in the cognitive behavioral and psychodynamic
rotations.

5 * Learning to Doctor in CBT

About a month into my fieldwork, I joined a group of psychiatry residents for a meeting of the rotation on cognitive behavioral therapy (CBT) for anxiety. At one point, Kelly, a social work trainee, asked her colleagues whether they had any experience with "GAD [generalized anxiety disorder] patients," people who experience persistent worries or fears that are out of proportion with their day-to-day lives.[1] Don (MSW), a midcareer social worker and skilled CBT clinician, offered that "with them you can do a lot of cognitive exposure," referring to a CBT technique. Damian (PGY-3) interjected, "Well, they're the patients that can do really well with SSRIs!"[2] "They've never been on medications," he continued, "and then I'll put them on something, and they come back loving me!" Amused, Kelly retorted, "Then I'll just send you all my patients!" Damian had yet to develop the epistemic generosity required to engage with his colleague's conundrum on CBT terms, approaching it instead as a skeptical psychiatrist. Still new to psychotherapy, he fell back on his pharmacological knowledge. His response, though confident, did not convince. To be recognized as competent in CBT, Damian would have to develop new doctoring skills.

In chapter 4, I showed the residents positioned as witnesses in their instructors' performances of psychotherapeutic expertise. Whether they observed experienced clinicians working with patients directly, glimpsed these experts' tacit knowledge in conversations, or heard them extol the merits of their own approaches, the residents were outsiders looking in. Yet becoming competent therapists required them to become insiders, and this chapter follows the residents as they do so in CBT. Competence in CBT was within relatively easier reach. This is partly because of its affinities with biopsychiatry, sharing a focus on symptoms and diagnoses, and on concrete tools and interventions aimed at mitigating patients' suffering. Unlike in psychodynamic psychotherapy where, as I will show in chapter 6, the residents had to learn entirely new ways to think about their patients, themselves, and the treatment relationship, their task was more bounded in CBT. Here, just as in biopsychiatry, their attention was trained on addressing their patients' conscious thoughts and behaviors with concrete tools—in this case, cognitive and behavioral instead of pharmacological.

Training was geared toward equipping the residents with just such pragmatic knowledge, unfolding during weekly two-hour meetings over six-month rotations. Not all residents participated in these rotations at the same time; the meetings involved subgroups of those who had expressed interest and received instructor permission to attend. In turn, these residents were mentored by clinicians who also trained social workers and psychologists and frequently found themselves in the company of these trainees. Individual supervision was done on an ad hoc basis, with the residents relying largely on group meetings to work through treatment conundrums. Finally, with the exception of CBT for children and adolescents, the residents were not required to conduct CBT treatments, though their instructors certainly encouraged them to do so. Instead, as I showed in chapter 3, the psychiatrists frequently opted to incorporate CBT techniques into medication management sessions.

Participating in psychotherapy rotations compelled the residents to actively engage in their own constitution as therapists. Practically, this meant learning therapeutic techniques and applying them with patients, delivering clinical case presentations, contributing to case discussions, and performing in role-plays. While the residents were familiar with case presentations and discussions from their earlier training, they did have to confront new expectations about the content of such exercises in CBT. As for role-plays, the residents were entirely new to this mode of apprenticeship. Role-plays, anthropologist E. Summerson Carr has pointed out, are "concertedly pragmatic exercises" that allow trainees to explore and develop conversational strategies in preparation for whatever patients bring up in sessions.[3] In CBT rotations, the manifest intent of such activities was to help novices work through interactional conundrums they might encounter during sessions. But the exercises also made visible the residents' abilities to think and act within a CBT framework, opening them up to examination, feedback, and self-reflection. Along with the conversations that followed, role-plays revealed the epistemic and professional friction the residents confronted, their doubts about the approach, and their struggles to overcome them.

It is worth noting here that whereas direct work with patients is an important element of gaining competence, it is not sufficient for managing the epistemic and professional frictions embedded in the residents' roles. Social scientists have long shown that novices' professional imaginaries are largely shaped by their interactions with peers and superiors.[4] As such,

I focus my analysis on the dynamics of psychotherapy group meetings because they stoked the frictions in the residents' roles and activated their skepticism, while also helping them to navigate these challenges.[5] In group discussions, the residents could learn new ways to doctor from their colleagues and instructors, share their struggles and doubts, and hear professional testimonials that together amounted to the collective management of skepticism.

This chapter traces the residents' journeys from skeptical and relatively ignorant outsiders to increasingly self-reflexive and competent CBT initiates. Though they do find themselves on somewhat familiar terrain, CBT still challenges the residents to think differently about their patients' problems and perform new roles as trainees. These frictions generate skepticism, and the first part of the chapter shows the residents struggling with their new epistemic mandate and working to establish their worth. Their dilemmas are especially pronounced during role-plays, and the second part of the chapter traces the efforts of one resident as he tries to inhabit a CBT doctoring role during one such exercise. Though he fumbles, the supportive presence of peers and instructors and the low stakes of the exercise itself make this a useful opportunity for experimenting with a new doctoring approach. The third part of the chapter illuminates the residents' increasing willingness to engage with CBT as insider participants, this time through self-reflection and self-work. In group discussions, the residents identify and address gaps between their biopsychiatric and CBT repertoires and are increasingly open to applying CBT tools to themselves. All the while, they signal their readiness and active cooperation in reshaping their doctoring practices. The chapter concludes with the residents' professional testimonials about the utility of the CBT techniques they are learning. As they share their successes, they also implicitly contribute to the collective management of skepticism.

Confronting Novicehood with Skepticism Early in CBT Training

The residents came up against the limitations of their existing knowledge early in their CBT training. Though they could build on their biopsychiatric repertoire of diagnoses and symptoms, they were also confronted by new ways of thinking about their patients' illnesses along with new interactional and role expectations. These frictions activated their skepticism, and the residents turned to their clinical experience to assert a modicum of professional worth. Yet commonalities between doctoring pharmacologically and doctoring in CBT helped ease their doubts, enabling a deeper engagement with the approach.

THE CHALLENGES OF THINKING WITH A CBT LENS

About a month into my fieldwork in the CBT for anxiety rotation, a case discussion revealed the residents' challenges with shifting from a biopsychiatric to a CBT framework. Draymond (PGY-3) began with a presentation of the case of Jessica, a patient he had recently met:

> OK, so she's a Caucasian woman, seventeen and a half years old, has been treated for ADHD [attention deficit hyperactivity disorder] and she then started complaining about depression—this is also the reason why she came in to see us, because she was suffering from depression over a breakup. But, when we saw her, we also saw that she has some anxiety: she scored high on the social anxiety scale. Specifically, she experiences anxiety before school and, because her mother works two jobs, she needs to take care of herself, so she drives herself to school. . . . She has social anxiety associated with school attendance, and she doesn't feel like she has enough friends.

Draymond included the key elements of a CBT case presentation—elements that overlapped with what he had already learned during his biopsychiatric training: he identified the patient's initial complaint ("depression"), another potential diagnosis ("social anxiety"), and the means by which he had reached it ("the social anxiety scale"). He momentarily set aside the patient's pharmaceutical treatment, signaling an opening toward thinking with CBT. Though he presented some telling information about Jessica's life circumstances and relationships—her working mother and her need to "take care of herself"—they were only of passing interest. What mattered more, Draymond knew, were the patient's thoughts and her actions in those contexts that she found most distressing: her "school attendance" and friendships.

Jeremy, the instructor in this orientation, quickly directed the residents' attention toward a CBT framework: "When we think about her, we should think about avoidances for exposure, thoughts for cognitive restructuring, and some social skills that she could learn." The experienced clinician zeroed in on the dimensions of the patient's illness that would be amenable to CBT intervention. The task for Draymond, Jeremy made clear, was to get a detailed and accurate account of his patient's idiosyncratic worries, thoughts, and behaviors so that he could begin to help her change them.

But Draymond did not have such information at the ready: "As we were talking to her, it was me and another med student, it was just a little hard to talk to her, to get her to tell us something specific. Her answers to our questions were really vague." The situation, the residents knew well, was not unusual. Patients are infrequently fully forthcoming about their illnesses, especially upon first meeting mental health care providers. But what made the patient's insufficient disclosure more challenging in this context was Draymond's own limited CBT repertoire. Jeremy tasked the group with figuring out what "cognitive restructuring" might look like for the patient. Doing this, I had come to learn, required a particular form of knowledge; namely, the ability to come up with plausible hypotheses about patients' thinking patterns.

Jeremy sought to work through such an exercise with Draymond and, when the resident admitted to not knowing much about his patient's thoughts, the instructor proposed matter-of-factly: "We'll just have to speculate."

> *Jeremy (Instructor)*: Could you imagine what she would have to say if you were to ask her about what she thinks during these scenarios?
> *Draymond (PGY-3)* [*channeling the patient*]: I'm bad at school and nobody likes me . . .
> *Jeremy*: OK, these are depressogenic thoughts.
> *Draymond*: OK, let me take another swing at this.
> [*Draymond offers another thought that Jeremy classifies as "depressogenic."*]
> *Jeremy*: That's OK. . . . Does she have or make any predictions? For example, would she say that if she talks to people, they will . . . laugh at her? Or maybe they will ignore her?

The resident could not distinguish between "depressogenic" thoughts and those that would have fit better with the "anxious patient" model Jeremy was trying to construct. "Predictions," the experienced clinician clarified, were more in line with a CBT treatment for anxiety—the focus of that rotation. Draymond's unsuccessful attempts at channeling his patient's anxious thoughts stemmed from the epistemic friction in his role. When he admitted to not having talked with his patient "about the thoughts" she was having "when experiencing social anxiety," the resident was simply acknowledging the difference between a typical psychiatric interview and the approach he was learning in CBT. Even though, Draymond explained, the residents and experienced CBT clinicians "on the depression team" had "talked about the interdigitation between depression and anxiety," he was not prepared to identify their differences (or overlaps) in patients' accounts. To successfully implement CBT, Draymond would have to become competent at just such a task.

Nevertheless, despite revealing his ignorance in CBT, Draymond could still turn to pharmacology to establish his professional worth: "The standard spiel I give people is that the medications will target both." He did not need to disentangle his patient's depressive and anxious thoughts to write a prescription that would treat her symptoms. The residents could always appeal to pharmaceutical know-how to show themselves as more than ignorant novices.

FRICTION AND ITS MANAGEMENT DURING ROLE-PLAYS

The residents' conundrums were heightened by their difficulties with role-plays. These exercises' manifest function was to help the residents develop new doctoring repertoires in low-stakes contexts. Occupying the role of therapist or patient, they could practice talking and thinking in a CBT framework. However, role-plays were also, inevitably, occasions for friction, illuminating disjunctures between the residents' existing professional repertoires and the approach they were learning. Though they could still be productive, these exchanges also illuminated the residents' reluctance to submit to the demands of CBT training.

During one of the initial meetings of the anxiety rotation, I witnessed a short role-play in which Don (MSW), taking the part of therapist, and Leah (PGY-3), that of patient, worked through a treatment problem she had brought up: how to speak with a patient who suffered from panic attacks and frequently came to the emergency room for fear of heart failure. Don, as the more experienced clinician, would be the therapist, modeling to Leah and her colleagues how they could talk with the patient. Leah would channel her own patient, a role that, theoretically, should have posed few problems.

> *Leah (PGY-3)/Patient*: I have chest pain when I get worked up about stuff and I know each year people drop dead from this . . .
>
> *Don (MSW)/Therapist*: I don't mean to be smart with you, but how many times have you had panic attacks over the last year?
>
> *Leah/Patient* [*steps out of the role and tries to remember her patient's complaint*]: Well, here I have to think like a clinician. . . . About two times a week, so about a hundred over the whole year. [*Steps back into the role.*] And every time I thought I would have a heart attack!
>
> *Don/Therapist*: And how many times did you have an actual heart attack?
>
> *Leah/Patient*: Zero, but I go to the hospital because it's always a possibility . . .
>
> *Don/Therapist*: Did you get a lot of tests done when you were there? Did the doctors ever give you any sense that a heart attack is in your future?
>
> [*Leah/Patient acknowledges that they had not, but expresses more worries about having a heart attack.*]
>
> *Don/Therapist*: So, OK, it could be a concern, but what do you think the chances are for a person of your health and age to have a heart attack?
>
> *Leah* [*steps out of the patient role*]: Well, let's see, I'm a white female in her late twenties, so I guess pretty slim.

> *Don/Therapist*: Would you like for me to tell you about my experience as a clinician? Here at the clinic we've seen thousands of patients with panic attacks and yet none have ever died of a heart attack. I wonder if, when you get these panic attacks you might remind yourself of some things: (1) that you had a hundred panic attacks but never a heart attack; (2) that we have seen thousands of patients here with panic attacks that have not had heart attacks; (3) that the doctors have also told you that you have nothing to worry about with respect to a heart attack.

Still early in her CBT training, Leah had trouble inhabiting the patient role and only reluctantly participated in the task. Not used to the premise and format of role-plays as training exercises, the residents initially approached them skeptically, resisting the demands of their roles and, at times, trying to end the exercise altogether. Leah stepped out of the patient role several times and had to "think like a clinician" to answer Don's questions. She did not seek to inject her performance with the kind of verisimilitude I would later see residents embracing. Don, more experienced, did not waver from being the therapist—a role he had inhabited many times, both in such exchanges and with actual patients. He conducted the exercise with the Socratic questioning approach I would come to recognize as an essential CBT interactive technique. He also channeled an appropriately authoritative persona, helping his partner along.

And while up to then Leah had been merely a reluctant and uncertain novice, not quite compelling as a CBT patient, toward the end of the exchange she found an opening to salvage her professional performance through skepticism. When Don suggested that the patient "remind" herself of three things when she gets "these panic attacks," Leah retorted without skipping a beat, "OK, but while I have a panic attack it's pretty hard to sit there and think about these things!" Occupying the role of patient had made available an unexpected avenue for the resident's doubts. Don was prepared: "OK, we will put these things on a note card and all you need to remember when you have a panic attack is to pull out the note card that reminds you of these three things."

At that moment, Leah's demeanor changed: "I really like the idea of pulling out a note card in case of emergency. A panic attack is an emotion emergency, so the card is 'in case of emergency, break glass,' or look at card!" The boundary between clinician and (role-play) patient seemed to vanish momentarily as Leah enthusiastically accepted Don's solution. Her skepticism, too, had diminished. The note card became one of the favorite tools for the residents in this rotation. It was a reminder of the affinities between CBT and pharmacology: whether they wrote a prescription or a note card, the residents could give their patients something concrete to help them outside sessions. For Leah, it was the difference between doubt and acceptance. Nevertheless, as helpful as it was, learning about such concrete tools was not all it took to quell the residents' skepticism toward CBT. Indeed, Leah's retort hinted at a deeper source of skepticism: would patients actually use the tools at their disposal? The residents' experiences working with patients who could not or would not follow treatments left them doubtful about the possibility of implementing CBT.

CLINICAL EXPERIENCE AS AN AVENUE FOR SKEPTICISM AND PROFESSIONAL WORTH

Clinical experience was a useful conduit of skepticism as the residents navigated the frictions in their therapeutic roles. It afforded them a compelling vantage point from which to assert their professional standing by doubting CBT's basic premise: that patients could actually put the approach into practice on their own. Early in the CBT for depression rotation, Robert introduced the trainees to David Burns's book *Feeling Good: The New Mood Therapy*. He told them that he routinely began treatments by asking patients to read the first three chapters of *Feeling Good* so that they could become familiar with the CBT model and some commonly used tools—for example, a depression checklist measuring symptoms and the list of "cognitive distortions." After reading the chapters themselves, the residents were left with some doubts. Aaron, a PGY-3 who had just begun CBT training, explained, "I was surprised at how hopeful [Dr. Burns] makes the first part of the book sound. I would be a little skeptical of that. You have to be a particular kind of person to be able to apply a [therapeutic] technique and for it to work." Aaron left implicit his belief that some, if not most, of his patients were not the "kind" who would be able to read the book and make it work. During a later meeting, he asked Robert:

> So, when you're referring to tools, 'cause that comes up a lot [in CBT, . . .] I feel like the thought record and other things like that, I feel like those are good things for us to change [patients'] cognition, but I don't see them as realistic to expect of the patients that every time they have a distressing situation they sit down and do a thought record. . . . So, are there specific tools that you can teach the patients? Like when they're doing the fortune-teller thing, what's the next step?

While Aaron's question could be dismissed as the novice's inexperience, it also showcased his effort at establishing his doctoring competence. Aaron was not questioning his own ability to implement CBT tools. He was, instead, doubting CBT's basic premise; namely, that patients would rely on its tools to work on themselves outside sessions.[6] To get better, patients needed to use the "thought record," the "daily activity schedule," the "worry exploration" worksheet, the "examining the evidence" worksheet, and other such forms in their day-to-day lives. Aaron doubted patients would indeed do so. Sanjay (PGY-3) echoed his colleague's stance, explaining that CBT exercises "seem really hard," especially for patients who are "really steeped in their depression."

The residents' skepticism did not go unaddressed. To ease their concerns, Robert appealed to his own clinical experience: "I actually do see the thought record as a tool, for [patients] to have it as a tool that they can choose to use, not just a therapy method. 'Cause I do remember patients who have used it." In turn, more experienced colleagues could offer similar reinforcement. After watching a video of a mock CBT session in which a depressed patient reflected on some of the positive aspects of caring for an aging parent, Turner (PGY-3) remarked, "I may just be a really poor therapist, but the degree of insight and willingness to recognize the positive [in a negative situation] is not in my experience what happens with my patients." Though prefaced with a hint of self-criticism, Turner's comment was typical in its questioning of CBT: "my patients," the resident contended, do not have the "insight" nor "willingness" to undertake the difficult task of reframing their problems in the language of CBT. Jason (PGY-4), a senior resident, responded, "I think it depends on the patient. [. . .] I've seen some patients who will go there at the beginning." The junior residents had yet to develop such professional memory.

Whereas Turner (PGY-3) spoke from the perspective of the psychiatrist who had spent most of his training helping very sick patients at the hospital, Jason (PGY-4), more advanced, appealed to his work with relatively healthier patients at the clinic. Both residents relied on clinical experience to assert their doctoring know-how, but they did so to different ends: for Turner, it was a conduit of skepticism, whereas for Jason, it made possible deeper engagement with CBT. In both cases, clinical experience helped solidify the residents' claims to competence.

Inhabiting CBT Roles

Role-plays were the residents' principal avenues for practicing CBT. In the company of peers and instructors, the residents could experiment with new doctoring methods, try out various interactional strategies, and work through the conundrums of putting CBT tools into practice. But, as Leah's experience (described earlier in the chapter) made clear, they could also be avenues for epistemic and professional friction. I turn here to an illustration of how residents could work through such friction with the support of peers and instructors. Help from these trusted partners, whether in the form of re-assurances or practical tips, validation or gentle correction, was essential to rendering the residents' skepticism toward the exercise, and toward the very possibility of doing CBT, into a productive platform for experimentation.

Halfway through the CBT for depression rotation, Robert announced early in the meeting that he would "like to [. . .] continue doing some role-play." We had spent several meetings already with these practical exercises and, that day, Robert announced with a smile, Sanjay (PGY-3), the resident who had avoided participation until then, could no longer do so. Turner (PGY-3) would be the patient, a role he had already practiced during a previous meeting. Robert instructed Sanjay: "So as he's talking, think about particular emotions he might be having, [ask him] what are the situations and what are the automatic thoughts. You don't have to formally say this is CBT, you can just start doing it, and just take an emotional episode and split it into situation and thoughts which may cause the feelings, and show [Turner] how to analyze that."

As a final encouragement, Robert playfully exhorted the resident: "Try to stay in role!" We had already heard Sanjay express his misgivings about the demands of role-play, and about being observed, earlier in the rotation. Sanjay did so again by way of response: "I just have such a hard time with role-playing! I don't know if it's performance anxiety . . ." As his thought trailed off, he shifted to face Turner on one side of the conference table.

Turner (PGY-3)/Patient: So, nice to meet you! "The reason I'm here today is 'cause I need refills for my meds . . ."
Sanjay (PGY-3)/Therapist [laughs, has trouble responding].
Turner [stepping out of his role]: That's what the patient told me!
Sanjay/Therapist [laughs and addresses the group]: It's a nervous laugh! [He returns to the role.] So what was Dr. Greer seeing you for?
Turner/Patient: I've had a lot of problems with alcohol recently! And I was in a detox program!
Sanjay/Therapist: So was Dr. Greer seeing you for detox?
Turner/Patient: It was kind of both, because I was depressed since 2007, and I was in jail for drunk driving, and while I was there my wife said don't bother coming back. . . . I've just been depressed since getting out of prison, I kept getting suicidal. . . . It's been really difficult . . . but I feel like there's a little bit of hope now, because of the detox, and living in a shelter!
Sanjay/Therapist: So it sounds like since you've had a lot of difficulties, you're still completely helpless . . . [Laughs, steps out of his role, and addresses the group.] Sorry, I'm trying to contain myself! [Collects himself and returns to his role.] So tell me a little bit more about your depression.

Turner/Patient: It feels like I just have nothing, I used to have a job, there's just nothing for me, and I never expected to be reduced to this! 'Cause now, I'm hopeless, I don't have a place to live . . .

Sanjay/Therapist: And that's an added challenge during this time, is being able to stay sober . . .

Turner/Patient: I don't think I'd be able to do it except that I want to keep my housing . . .

The role-play got off to a rocky start. It was difficult for Sanjay to "stay in the role," as Robert had anticipated. Yet Sanjay also tried to maintain his credibility with his colleagues and instructor. His explanation that his was "nervous" laughter was meant to dispel any misinterpretations that he might have been laughing at Turner or the exercise itself. To be fair, Turner himself was injecting a bit more conviction into the role than I had seen other residents do in the past. His declarative statements verged on earnestness, making me wonder whether he was actually trying to make his colleague's job a little bit harder. It would soon become clear, though, that Turner was walking the fine line between offering Sanjay support and infusing his own role with authenticity.

Up to this point, their interaction had not been CBT specific, but Sanjay was able to collect himself and turn toward the task at hand:

Sanjay/Therapist: It sounds like your depression has been caused by your situation, and you also see things in a negative light.

The statement set the stage for a more explicit CBT conversation focused on Turner-qua-patient's "negative" thoughts and the situations that caused them. On cue, Turner responded:

Turner/Patient: Yeah, I feel like I shouldn't be here right now!

Sanjay/Therapist: What do you mean by that?

Turner/Patient: I used to have a job, and a house, I never thought I would be in jail . . .

Sanjay/Therapist: So before that, did you feel depressed?

Turner/Patient: A little bit [. . .] when my parents died, my brother died . . .

Sanjay/Therapist: What other things were going on at that time?

Turner/Patient: My life was pretty simple, I worked construction. . . . There wasn't a whole lot, my life was kind of empty, 'cause when my family members died, it's like, what's left?

Sanjay/Therapist: So I'm hearing a couple of things, and it seems like sometimes when things get hard, it's difficult to see the reason for continuing on . . .

Sanjay and Turner were getting into a rhythm as CBT therapist and patient. Turner seemed to inhabit his role with ease. Without the burden of nervous laughter, Sanjay's performance, too, offered glimpses of his doctoring skills. He asked open-ended questions that created opportunities for Turner's disclosure and reoriented the discussion again toward CBT: "when things get hard, it's difficult to see the reason for continuing on." Translated into CBT terms, Sanjay was explaining that tough situations cloud patients' thinking and worsen their feelings. He was on his way to salvaging his performance.

But, instead of identifying such a situation and working with Turner in the manner that Robert had advised, Sanjay retreated from the task of implementing CBT. Instead, he fell back on his biopsychiatric repertoire, drawing Turner as patient into a discussion of his illness history and life circumstances. Yet even as his CBT skills were receding from view, Sanjay's competence in setting a collaborative tone came through: as Turner disclosed bits of his troubles and feelings in the patient role, Sanjay repeated and summarized them, employing a typical therapeutic strategy for strengthening the treatment relationship. He also asked questions that invited further elaboration. At one point, when Turner-qua-patient disclosed that he had been thinking about suicide almost daily in recent weeks, Sanjay reflected his feelings:

Sanjay/Therapist: So it sounds like, if I'm understanding you correctly, it sounds like things haven't been going very well, like you're saying a lot of things like things are hopeless . . . you certainly feel that way? In those times, did you really feel like literally there is no hope?

Turner/Patient: Well, people here have been really nice, and that gives me some hope. . . . I'm actually getting some medical care . . .

Sanjay/Therapist: So things weren't, didn't seem to be so hopeless . . .

Turner/Patient: Yeah, it surprises me that there are still people there that still care . . .

Sanjay/Therapist: Do you think that may be the case with some other things too?

Turner/Patient: Like I'm not completely worthless?

Sanjay/Therapist: Yeah. . . . So, is that something you might be interested in talking a little bit more about? How you feel about things that make you feel so down as compared to how things are?

Turner knew what was expected of him as a patient in a CBT role-play. In offering such a compelling performance, he was establishing his own competence in the approach. He even helped Sanjay along in moments when he seemed to lose the thread, offering "I'm not completely worthless" as a concrete counterpoint to the more negative thoughts he had expressed earlier in the role-play. This, too, was a typical CBT move, but one that therapists were typically expected to help their patients make. The comment set Sanjay up for a return to conducting a CBT intervention, proposing that they compare "how things are" with how the patient "feels[s] about things." To that invitation, Turner offered an enthusiastic "Definitely!" and explained, "I'm willing to do anything now, 'cause I'm just trying to stay sober." Though an actual patient may have been less enthusiastic at the prospect of self-work, Turner was trying to balance the demands of his role with his desire to help out his colleague. Sanjay seemed ready to begin doing CBT rather than simply priming the patient for it.

> *Sanjay/Therapist:* But it sounds like a lot of the day you spend thinking about what you've lost. . . . One of the things that we know about depression is that, we know that how you feel can really affect how you think about something and how you behave. . . . And what we know about depression is that it works the other way too: where how you think about things and how you do things affects the way you felt about it too. . . . Have you ever felt like you went somewhere where you didn't really want to go and still had a good time?
>
> *Turner/Patient:* Well, I didn't think that I could get as far as I have without drinking . . .
>
> *Sanjay/Therapist:* So that's a similar thing. . . . So if you're spending all day thinking about how hopeless and worthless you are, then that will affect how you think about things. . . . But sometimes our brains jump ahead of us and distort reality. [*Sanjay hands Turner the list of "cognitive distortions."*] Do any of these things on the list seem like you do them?
>
> *Turner/Patient:* Maybe catastrophizing. . . . But my life *is* really bad . . .
>
> *Sanjay/Therapist:* One of the things that we can talk about is thinking that everything is hopeless. . . . How do you feel about that?

Somewhat awkwardly, Sanjay brought the conversation to the point where he could implement a CBT technique. He proceeded with care, setting up the collaboration and asking the patient whether he would be willing to examine his thought that "everything is hopeless"—a key part of doctoring in CBT. He then gave Turner a list of "cognitive distortions" and asked him to identify which one applied to his own thinking. And while Turner as patient seemed willing to work in this vein, identifying "catastrophizing" as a possible "distortion" he engaged in, he also stopped being as accommodating. In response to Sanjay's question, Turner offered a reminder that, outside the conference room, patients are less easygoing:

> *Turner/Patient*: Well, usually I can't really think that much when I feel that way. . . . I just think about why is my life so miserable, and it doesn't seem like my life is worth living . . .

At this point, the role-play stopped abruptly as Sanjay admitted, "All right, I'm actually a little bit lost right now." Robert was ready with practical advice: "You can talk about his view of himself as worthless. So see if he can see that it's not helpful to think that he's worthless because it makes him more depressed, and also see if there's evidence to the contrary." Turner had thrown a wrench into Sanjay's performance, but Robert was there to assist. After the short interlude, the role-play continued, with Turner returning to his earlier, more helpful, stance.

> *Turner/Patient*: I do feel worthless! I feel like somebody else would in my situation: Like my neighbors still live in their homes and have a job, and so I feel like a complete loser . . .
> *Sanjay/Therapist*: So do you feel like you tell that to yourself a lot?
> *Turner/Patient*: Yeah . . . and it makes me feel horrible, like I just wanna kill myself!
> *Sanjay/Therapist*: So it sounds like those thoughts are feeding back into the depression.

Robert interrupted with affirmation: "So you got him to the point where he is seeing that those thoughts are feeding back into the depression." Sanjay was on the right track:

> *Sanjay/Therapist*: Let's try and break this down. . . . So you gave some reasons for why you feel worthless. Can you think of anything positive that's happened in the last couple of months?
> *Turner/Patient*: The [quitting] drinking definitely! And now I have a place to live and I've been trying to get a job . . .
> *Sanjay/Therapist*: So in that sense you are headed in a positive direction. . . . How does that make you feel?
> *Turner/Patient*: It makes me feel better . . .

Sanjay had just completed a short CBT intervention: he had not only explained that the patient's thinking can shape his feelings but had also challenged his belief that he was "worthless." The exchange offered a glimpse of his budding competence in this doctoring approach. But the role-play was about to take yet another turn that would reveal Sanjay's novicehood and necessitate face-saving maneuvers:[7]

Sanjay/Therapist: So it sounds like there are some parts where you feel bad . . .

Turner/Patient [interjects, heartfelt]: Do you think I'm worthless, doctor?

Sanjay/Therapist [laughing]: I think that anybody who has managed to get through what you've gone through is not worthless.

At this point, Sanjay, Turner, and Robert all burst out laughing. Sanjay had a difficult time stepping back into the role and asserted amid laughter: "I'm actually really, really good with patients, I promise! I just can't, I warned you!" The comment, intended to defend his professionalism, opened the door for a mini–CBT intervention. Robert immediately picked up the cognitive "distortion" and pushed back on the resident's stance: "Now, is it really true that you can't, or . . ." He did not have to complete his sentence, as Sanjay interjected, "It's just very challenging, but not impossible!" Sanjay recovered some of his doctoring competence by accepting Robert's reframing and going along with it as in a typical CBT exchange. He then turned to his colleague: "I'm sorry, Turner, it's just that you're so good at being in that role! I'm sorry . . ." With mock seriousness, Turner responded, "Well, you told me that I'm not worthless and I feel a little bit better!" This sent Sanjay into another bout of laughter, to which he remarked, "I'm sorry, I just can't help it!"—only to immediately correct himself: "I *can* help it, it's just difficult!"

After everyone regained their composure, the role-play proceeded with Sanjay and Turner continuing to identify aspects of the patient's life that would demonstrate his worth rather than worthlessness. Robert again interrupted to suggest "things to try out." All were practical strategies: "Have [the patient] think of a best friend and explore if his best friend would have gone through what he's gone through, would he think that he was worthless"; or ask the patient whether he thought "that people who make mistakes" are "worthless." But, when Robert asked, "Why don't you try that?" Sanjay exclaimed, "I was so excited about being done!" Picking up on the resident's reluctance, Robert offered to "take over" and give him some "relief." But Sanjay demurred: "No, I can do it, but I need to control my laughter!" Not willing to admit failure, Sanjay was committed to seeing the performance through.

As they implemented Robert's suggestions in the final part of the role-play, Turner reassumed his role as a good patient while Sanjay successfully guided him through the "think of a best friend" exercise. When Turner cooperatively stated, "I've never thought about it that way, but maybe I've been a little bit unfair to myself," Sanjay stepped out of the role to showcase his CBT thinking: "OK, so from here I would just be merging with the thing I was doing before, about the cognitive distortions." Robert affirmed and offered further advice about how he could "put a finer point on" how unrealistic the patient's self-judgments were. He also provided an entirely different approach to the same problem, taking over the role-play and briefly performing the therapist role with Turner as the patient.

At last, Robert declared the exercise over: "All right, we can stop now! Yaaay, you did it! It was only difficult because of the laughing!" At roughly thirty minutes, the role-play was the longest I had witnessed, partly because of Sanjay's difficulties staying in the role and partly because of his troubles inhabiting a competent version of a CBT therapist. After the resident repeated that he's "good with patients," Robert reassured him that "we're not generalizing to your experiences with patients!" Turner too offered his own form of validation: "It was interesting being the patient." He added, "You often wonder, when you're giving advice, how that's perceived." Turner was acknowledging some of the conundrums of helping patients with tools he and his colleagues did not yet feel competent using. But, Turner reflected, the experience of playing the patient taught him that "if you feel like someone is being helpful and wants to help, you probably are open to a broad range of advice." "Patients probably don't obsess over whether it's right or not," he surmised, implicitly offering Sanjay his own form of reassurance.

While Sanjay's difficulties inhabiting the role of therapist manifested themselves in his anxiety around the performance, his troubles were indicative of a fundamental dilemma all residents confronted: how to establish their doctoring worth in situations that positioned them as ignorant novices. Role-play offered the residents opportunities to practice CBT talk and techniques. Although failure was less consequential in this context—in the sense that no actual patients were involved—it was not insignificant. The residents wanted to do well—both because they were doctors eager to establish their professional capabilities and because role-plays were conduits of implicit assessment by peers and, more important, instructors. Though he had offered constructive criticism during the exercise itself, Robert praised Sanjay after his performance for doing "a good job of showing empathy and building an alliance before doing the technical CBT stuff." This was not just ceremonial recognition. Robert had long stressed the importance of collaboration, and Sanjay had indeed set such a tone in the role-play. In praising the resident's approach, Robert affirmed his incipient therapeutic skill.

Developing Self-Reflexivity on the Path to Competence

As they began to engage with CBT more extensively, the residents became increasingly aware of their shortcomings in the approach. I took this awareness, along with their efforts at redressing gaps in their knowledge, as a mark of their transition from outsiders to ready and engaged participants in learning CBT. Two simultaneous processes signaled this shift. On the one hand, they became more reflective about gaps between their biopsychiatric doctoring practices and what they were expected to do in CBT. On the other hand, they also became more willing and adept at applying CBT tools to their personal lives.

ACKNOWLEDGING AND ADDRESSING GAPS BETWEEN BIOPSYCHIATRIC AND CBT DOCTORING

About two months into the CBT for depression rotation, Robert asked the residents whether "anybody [has] anything to report." Aaron (PGY-3) shared a recent attempt at using a CBT tool: "I did a thought record, but I'm not sure I did it the right way." He went on, "The patient said his main fear is that he's gonna die early, and then I put that as the event and then when I asked him what he thinks about, he said that he's worried about killing himself." Aaron admitted, "I don't think I used the thought record correctly." Even as he acknowledged his novice ignorance, Aaron immediately offered, "I should have tried to elicit some situation that elicits [those] thoughts." By disclosing his mistake and offering a solution, he demonstrated his willingness to engage with CBT and projected his growing knowledge—if not yet practical competence—of its techniques.

Aaron was not alone in sharing his conundrums and his growing insights with the group. Sanjay (PGY-3) had his own difficulties:

> [The patient] says, "I have ten thoughts a day that make me anxious" and then, when I asked her about it, she said that she doesn't want to think about them because she's worried that if she starts processing them, she'll feel an overwhelming anxiety and feel really depressed! I spent a lot of time telling her that that was a cognitive distortion rather than eliciting that from her.

Akin to Aaron, Sanjay could identify his CBT mistake: he "told" his patient that her thinking was distorted "rather than eliciting that from her." He had fallen back on his medical habits, diagnosing the patient's problem rather than engaging her in self-examination. But by disclosing his error, the resident did more than simply position himself as a CBT novice. He, too, was revealing his incipient psychotherapeutic abilities. Even though he had failed to collaborate with his patient, he could still demonstrate a modicum of CBT knowledge. His confession, akin to Aaron's, showcased a willingness to reflect on and reshape his doctoring repertoire. And while this signaled a lessening in the residents' skepticism toward doctoring without drugs, achieving competence in this approach required them to practice CBT not simply with their patients but also on themselves.

INTERNALIZING CBT THROUGH SELF-WORK

Sanjay's (PGY-3) self-work went beyond his analysis of the treatment misstep he shared with his colleagues. After discussing the case for several minutes, the resident jokingly reflected, "I have a lot of anxiety about . . ." He left the thought unfinished, only to reformulate it: "I have a cognitive distortion about how I will do with this therapy." While his initial statement hinted at his novicehood and the worries associated with it, Sanjay distanced himself from this position and the feelings associated with it by employing a core CBT concept, cognitive distortion. Robert responded as an expert CBT clinician would, proposing a counterfactual: "What would it be like if things didn't go well in this session?" He made Sanjay's concerns concrete and identified a situation—his next session with his patient—where they could focus the "intervention." Sanjay offered, "I'm catastrophizing," referring to a common cognitive distortion. Robert offered an alternative: "It could be fortune-telling, that you know you're not gonna do well." He did not wait for Sanjay to respond, simply offering a typical CBT retort— "What's the likelihood with that?"—followed by validation: "I appreciate you sharing with us your own anxiety, and of course that is the best place to start: working on our own anxieties and predictions." Sanjay laughingly agreed: "Oh, I was a complete basket case when I started out here!"

Though Sanjay's final admission was uncommon, it hinted at an important aspect of psychotherapeutic training: working on oneself and developing self-reflexivity. As I show in chapter 6, in psychodynamic training the residents were frequently reminded how consequential self-knowledge is to building and understanding therapeutic relationships with patients. In CBT, self-reflexivity took on less weighted meaning. Here, self-awareness and self-work were posited as conduits for learning the intervention's tools, only indirectly constitutive of successful treatments. To be clear, not all the residents were as receptive as Sanjay to this dimension of training.

Nora, the social worker and respected therapist who trained the residents in dialectical behavior therapy (DBT), was apt to engage novices in self-work exercises. During the first meeting of the DBT rotation, Nora explained to the group, including seven residents (a mix of PGY-3s and PGY-4s): "I want you to have some of the concepts, strategies, that will allow you to go into a room with someone who will rip your head out one day and love you the next." The key to developing this ability, she explained, was to work on themselves with DBT tools. Nora stressed, "With DBT, we teach our patients skills and we learn those skills ourselves." Cedric (PGY-3), new to psychotherapy training, remarked on how unusual Nora's appeal to "practice what we preach" was. Not wishing to appear contrary, he affirmed that "it's useful" because "before we can ask a patient to get insight and engage in these activities, we should have some insight about it ourselves." Though conciliatory, Cedric's remark betrayed his doubts about the requirements made of him as a novice in DBT. The resident was becoming increasingly aware of the contradictions he would have to navigate as he began his psychotherapy training.

Nora sought to quiet the residents' concerns by portraying the process of self-work as unfolding organically: "It ends up, 'That's for the patient but, oh yeah, I used that with my wife, or I used that with my kid, and it worked.'" Yet it soon became clear that she did not leave self-reflexivity to chance. The residents were to come to group meetings prepared to discuss how they had applied DBT skills either in their work with patients or in their own lives. For example, early in the very next meeting, Nora wanted the group to review the skills of "mindfulness."[8] As the residents hesitantly worked through the answers, the following exchange ensued:

Octavia (PGY-3): Is it the thing about "observe"?
Nora (Instructor): How would you apply "observe" to "wise mind"?
Vivya (PGY-3): Is it observe without making judgments . . .
Nora: You have to observe in order to know what your emotion is. . . . Like right now, what are you feeling? What are you feeling, Octavia?
Octavia: [*Pause*] I could not think of an emotion. . . . Comfortable, glad . . .
[*Nora turns toward the class, seeking other contributions.*]
Cedric (PGY-3): I feel guilty, 'cause I was late . . .
Jarvis (PGY-4): I'm happy. . . .
Mariana (Ethnographer): Overwhelmed . . .
Nora: So you see how you had to stop and observe. . . . You need to teach your patients to observe, and you also need to learn how to do that. . . . You're observing all kinds of things about your patients all the time—how they look, how they feel . . . One of the things that we need to work on more is observing *our* emotional state.

The residents were not used to discussing their feelings in such formal professional settings (neither was I). Sandra, a psychiatrist who completed her residency during my time at Shorewood, told me that, before the psychotherapy rotations, doctors' and nurses' own emotions "would get talked about in rounds on the inpatient unit [at the hospital] sometimes, like if the unit was getting really stressed out or something, because the patient was splitting and [the staff] were getting angry at the patient, then we would talk about it." Outside such circumstances, as Nora rightly noted, the residents focused their efforts on identifying and understanding patients' emotions while largely ignoring their own. In psychotherapy they would have to turn the lens toward themselves. For the residents, this meant making the task of self-awareness a routine part of learning a new way to doctor.

Instructors rarely missed a chance at routinizing such self-reflexivity. When Jason (PGY-4) exclaimed that he felt "way too happy that my 5:00 p.m. patient canceled!" Robert retorted:

> Robert (Instructor) [amused]: I have an interpretation about that: you wanted to go home early and start your weekend! [Laughs.]
> Jason (PGY-4) [continues laughing]: I shouldn't be happy about that; it makes me a bad doctor!
> Robert [jokingly]: Aahh, cognitive distortion! Grist for the mill!

As Robert playfully adopted a psychodynamic stance with "I have an interpretation about that," he rejected the depth psychological approach in favor of CBT's emphasis on conscious meaning. Unlike in psychodynamic psychotherapy, where Jason's happiness would have been mined for meaning in light of his relationship with his patient, in CBT it was simply taken as his relief at the weekend's arrival. But, when Jason worried that his feeling made him a "bad doctor," he also opened the door for CBT intervention. Wittingly or not, he became a CBT object: his thought rendered into a cognitive distortion, it was "grist for the mill" of self-tuning with the aid of CBT techniques.

I came to view such exchanges in CBT and DBT as particularly effective at getting residents to internalize, and even accept, the tenets of these approaches. Though these discussions seemed to position them in roles akin to patients, the residents were not compelled to give up professional control. Unlike the focus on the residents' inner lives in psychodynamic supervision, which, as I showed in chapter 3, threatened their sense of themselves as professionals, self-work in CBT and DBT had fewer such reverberations. Jason was not simply subject to a CBT intervention. He was also the agent of the kind of self-tuning Robert encouraged. The approach offered the residents a way to work on themselves without the complications of becoming patients—a necessary, but frequently resisted, part of the kind of self-reflexivity encouraged in psychotherapy training.[9] Moreover, unlike in their relationships with psychoanalytic supervisors, such exchanges in CBT offered the residents more control over the personal-professional boundary. They created a path for the residents to broaden their skill set by working on themselves and doing so without risking too much exposure of their personal lives and a possible loss of face.

Offering Professional Testimonials and Managing Skepticism Collectively

CBT offered the residents an easier path toward success. They found its tools practicable in a variety of settings and sometimes experienced swift success with their application. And, when they shared their positive experiences with their peers, the residents offered what I came to think of as professional testimonials about the utility of the approach. Thus shoring up CBT's legitimacy, they also implicitly contributed to the collective management of skepticism.

Early in the CBT for depression rotation, I was surprised to hear some of the junior residents praising its tools even as they had little knowledge of them and their application. During their third meeting together, Sanjay (PGY-3) asked Robert whether he had any experience applying CBT "in an acute short-term setting, like the inpatient unit." Sanjay and the other two PGY-3s in the group had completed their inpatient rotations less than a month before, and the hospital loomed large in their professional imaginaries. Robert admitted that he had not "worked with inpatients in a long time," but he assured the residents that there are "studies" and "books" on integrating CBT in such contexts. Turner (PGY-3) chimed in, "I think that one of the most helpful things [you taught us] was progressive muscle relaxation and deep breathing. Those are extremely useful in a short-term setting even in, like, PES [psychiatric emergency services]." Mere weeks into CBT training, Turner could already identify techniques that he could use when psychiatric drugs were not enough.

As the residents began to develop competence in CBT, they could share practical successes with their colleagues, offering the kind of professional testimonials that were an implicit but essential part in the management of skepticism. Recall Damian (PGY-3), who, in the chapter's opening, evaded Kelly's question about a CBT treatment by referring to the effectiveness of SSRIs instead. Nearly three months later, Damian adopted a different stance. He began by asking his colleagues for help with a patient he had been treating for "three or four months." He explained, "She's a nineteen-year-old girl diagnosed with OCD" who had been "having a lot of intrusive thoughts" that caused her to engage in "compulsive praying" that amounted to "three hours a day." The patient had come to the clinic, the resident continued, "at the desperate cries of her therapist, for the OCD symptoms. [. . .] She was hoping that we'd have a medication that we could give her, and it [the OCD] would go away."

Damian did initially turn to his psychiatric toolkit. "We tried Celexa," he explained, but "she actually got more depressed on that. Went over to Zoloft and that's helped a lot of her general anxiety stuff, but it's not really touching her OCD stuff."[10] The resident had run out of pharmaceutical options. But he was also becoming more knowledgeable about CBT treatments for OCD. He decided to change course, "trying to sell [the patient] on the idea that, OCD, you can't think your way out of it, it's gotta be exposure, [and] here's how we can do it." No longer the skeptic, the resident had to undo his patient's doubts as well. This was no easy task: she was convinced of the necessity of striving for perfection through prayer, and she had also taken to researching psychiatric drugs and asking her psychiatrist, Damian, to prescribe them.[11] In turning to the group with this conundrum, Damian admitted to the limitations of his pharmaceutical tools and demonstrated his newfound belief in the usefulness of CBT.

Damian's experience was not unique. The residents were well aware of pharmacology's limitations across a range of diagnoses. Early in the CBT for depression rotation, Turner (PGY-3) admitted that "with antidepressants" he can "see [patients] bouncing back to a lower level of depression." But, he continued, "it seems that that initial enthusiasm is not the long-lasting change that you're looking for." Still new to psychotherapy training at the time, Turner admitted to not knowing "what to do in response to that." Training in talk and behavioral interventions would prepare him and his colleagues to fill gaps in their clinical knowledge and be better able to help patients. At a later meeting in the CBT rotation, Turner would showcase his growing competence: when he worked with patients for whom "medication is not indicated" but who still "want you to give them something," he could "just give them a [CBT] handout." Knowledgeable about the tools and skills that CBT had to offer, the resident was better equipped to care for patients. He was also well positioned to voice the kind of testimonial about the usefulness of CBT that might resonate with a more skeptical colleague.

Sanjay's skills, too, had improved, as had his confidence in his CBT doctoring abilities. At the end of the six months in the CBT rotation, Sanjay (PGY-3) shared, "I think last year [PGY-2], if I saw a patient at the hospital who was anxious or upset, I don't think I had any real idea about what to do. Now, I think I have a way to deal with that." When medications could not help, Sanjay could turn to CBT tools to "deal" with patients' feelings. This was not simply abstract talk. A little more than a month prior, Sanjay

(PGY-3) had told the group that he had encouraged one of the patients he treated with medications to also participate in a CBT therapy group at the clinic. The patient "seemed to get a pretty good benefit out of it." In fact, Sanjay emphatically declared, the patient had "looked a lot brighter and a lot better!" after he had attended the group. "I've just been emphasizing to him," the resident explained, "that we really want to replace the Ativan with CBT."[12] After spending a few months learning CBT, Sanjay's skepticism toward it softened, giving way to competence and, sometimes, conviction.

The residents' clinical experience could help them demonstrate their skills, this time in psychotherapy. And while earlier on such appeals lent themselves to expressions of doubt, later in their psychotherapy training the residents appealed to treatment experiences to share their conviction. In CBT for anxiety, Draymond (PGY-3) did just this. He had been working with a patient who had "a fear of driving," especially, the resident explained, "with fishtailing," losing control over a car as its rear wheels skid sideways in slippery road conditions. They had been working together on "some doughnuts in the parking lot"—the behavioral component of a CBT treatment for such fears. The exercises, the resident shared, "did help her with her fishtailing [fears]." Draymond confessed to the group that he "was surprised by that," immediately clarifying, "I did not reveal my surprise to her that my suggestions worked!" To his patient, Draymond was the competent doctor, confident in his treatment "suggestions." His doubts were for his colleagues' ears only. His success—surprising to him, but not to the experienced CBT clinicians who trained him—helped ease his, and possibly his colleagues', skepticism.

Conclusion

Early on, the residents approached CBT with the confidence and know-how of psychiatrists who could identify their patients' symptoms and treat them with pharmaceuticals. CBT's emphasis on concrete tools and delimited interventions placed them on familiar terrain. However, while this emphasis diminished some of the contradictions inherent in the residents' roles, it did not resolve them. The residents still had to face the professional and epistemic frictions of learning a new way to doctor. They had to confront anew the ignorance and subjection associated with being novices and to learn how to think beyond symptoms and diagnoses. They had to master the tools of CBT and develop strategies for using them with often skeptical patients.

This required the residents to work through their own skepticism. They took little issue with CBT interventions themselves. Instead, they doubted

CBT's basic assumption that patients could and would apply CBT techniques in their own lives. Clinical experience served them well in such displays of skepticism. When questioning a CBT intervention, the residents turned to versions of what became a familiar trope: "my" patients won't do it, won't buy it, or can't do it. Patients' voices and perspectives—as channeled by the residents themselves—were powerful tools in the psychiatrists' displays of professional competence. They lent themselves to declarations of skepticism or of success, as the occasion merited.

However, in psychotherapy group meetings, the residents were compelled to actively participate in the process of acquiring new doctoring tools, and role-plays were particularly productive in this respect. During such exercises, the residents could try out CBT "provisional selves," to borrow organizational scholar Herminia Ibarra's concept.[13] They could temporarily inhabit identities as therapists or patients, channeling interactional, conversational, and affective dispositions as required by the role. Doing so amounted to more than a practical accomplishment. Fundamentally, role-plays were, to quote E. Summerson Carr, "opportunities for participants to analyze *themselves*" (emphasis in original).[14] Through a combination of self-examination and feedback from the group, the residents could identify their doctoring strengths and troubleshoot their difficulties.

As they became more willing to engage with CBT on its own terms, the residents' skepticism took on a more productive and less defensive valence. In turn, trying out CBT interventions became both a professional and a personal project. Professionally, the residents grappled with the conundrums of novicehood in the company of peers and instructors, becoming increasingly aware of disjunctures between doctoring in biopsychiatry and doctoring in CBT. Yet as they began to reflect on their shortcomings as CBT practitioners, they also started to develop and showcase their growing knowledge of CBT itself. Such self-reflexivity was a stepping stone in the residents' shift from being dedicated biopsychiatrists to adopting more flexible doctoring roles.

The process was helped along by the kind of self-work that CBT instructors sought to routinize. Attention to one's own inner life, the instructors made clear, was a pragmatic means for the residents to practice the new techniques they were learning. Applying CBT tools to themselves deepened the residents' self-awareness, an essential ingredient in their journeys from skeptics to competent initiates. The exercises naturalized CBT tools and techniques, making them part of the residents' personal and professional repertoires of action. This self-work, alongside role-play, helped them shift from keeping CBT at arm's length to participating in their socialization in this epistemic culture.

In a community where much expert work happens behind closed doors, group settings opened the residents' skills up to examination and feedback. Case presentations, discussions, and role-play could ease the residents' defensive skepticism and foster their competence. With peers and instructors, they could discuss their conundrums, try out solutions, and reflect on themselves. In turn, the group offered validation and recognition alongside necessary corrections. The mutual support the residents gave one another, alongside the reinforcement they received from instructors, was essential to the collective management of skepticism and to fostering the residents' competence in new ways to doctor.

6 * Learning to Doctor Psychodynamically

Psychodynamic training posed the residents their most difficult challenges. Cognitive behavioral therapy (CBT) drew them in with its affinities with biopsychiatry, but there were few such affordances in psychodynamic psychotherapy. Here, the epistemic and professional frictions in the residents' roles were heightened, and their journeys from skepticism to competence more fraught and protracted. Nevertheless, with time, support, and opportunities to reflect on and experiment with this new approach, the residents did transition from skeptical outsiders to able participants in their constitution as psychodynamic initiates.

One afternoon about halfway through the residency year, I attended a meeting in the psychodynamic rotation during which Kai (PGY-4) delivered a case presentation. Kai had come prepared: he had several typed-up pages of therapy notes in front of him and read carefully from them, pausing to give his colleagues and the instructors, Terry and Patricia, contextual explanations. I was impressed with the accuracy and detail of his well-crafted *process notes*—the transcripts of therapy sessions that serve as the foundation for training in psychodynamic psychotherapy. But, during a break in Kai's presentation, Vinit (PGY-4) asked, "Kai, did you or your supervisor ever feel that [the patient] was a bad candidate for psychotherapy?" Vinit's question was motivated by his colleague's lengthy description of his patient's difficulties reflecting on his life and talking about his emotions. "My supervisor never thought that he was a bad candidate," Kai clarified. Lucas (PGY-3) jumped in: "I'm laughing because we share the same supervisor and I don't think he would say *anybody* is a bad person for psychodynamic therapy!" Vinit insisted: "I asked that because I wonder what a bad candidate for psychodynamic therapy would look like."

Vinit's skepticism stemmed partly from working with a patient who, akin to Kai's, had trouble talking about her inner life. His doubts were heightened by his biopsychiatric socialization and its emphasis on classifying patients into diagnostic and treatment categories. To him, the patient seemed ill suited to psychodynamic psychotherapy, an approach that partly depends on a willingness and ability to talk about feelings and relationships. And while Lucas's comment affirmed Kai's response, his laughter hinted at his own implicit skepticism toward their psychoanalytic supervisor's encompassing take on the applicability of the psychodynamic approach. In different ways, the two residents were signaling their doubts. Terry, the psychoanalyst and psychiatrist who co-led the rotation, interjected, addressing their doubts head-on: "I think there are two points to that: the manifest and latent content. The manifest content maybe didn't make [the patient] look shrinkable, being so concrete, but the latent part is that he was clearly interested in working on himself." Terry affirmed the supervisor's perspective and implicitly validated Kai's own trust.

Kai himself needed no further convincing. His case presentation and process notes made clear that, despite ongoing difficulties, his patient, Carl, had come to entrust him with significant parts of his life. They had formed a strong relationship that enabled Carl to talk about his emotions, his relationships, and his troubles. Kai too had come to think of his patient's problems less in terms of symptoms and more as functions of inner conflicts that manifested themselves in his relationships, particularly those with his wife and son. The resident had become increasingly attuned to his patient's desire for closeness and intimacy and spoke eloquently about how these desires manifested themselves in the therapeutic relationship. He also reflected on his own role in their interpersonal dynamic. During the case presentation, Kai emerged as a capable psychodynamic initiate, showcasing his competence in the approach.

In chapter 5, I showed how the residents transitioned from skeptical outsiders to ready and able participants in CBT. In this chapter, I illustrate the parallel, if more challenging, process in psychodynamic training. The following pages show the residents beginning to inhabit psychodynamic doctoring roles in clinical case presentations and discussions. Early on, they are reluctant to do so. Still rooted in biological psychiatry, they rely on their existing tool kit of symptoms and medication effects but find it falling short as they must think about their patients psychodynamically. The first part of the chapter illuminates the residents' struggles and shows them turning to skepticism to establish a sense of worth. But, with time, they begin to engage with psychodynamic psychotherapy on its own terms, and the second part of the chapter shows them reckoning with the distinct contours of psychodynamic doctoring roles and developing increasing facility with such roles through self-reflexivity. In the final part of the chapter I turn my attention to the senior residents' professional testimonials and their participation in the collective management of doubt. More experienced and less skeptical, advanced residents share their therapeutic successes by showcasing both their patients' and their own deepening self-insight. Their accounts, in turn, are powerful reminders to their more skeptical colleagues of the productivity and benefits of working psychodynamically.

Friction and Skepticism Early in Psychodynamic Training

Clinical case presentations and discussions were ubiquitous in the psychodynamic rotation, favored by Terry and fellow instructor Patricia over dialogue about psychoanalytic theories or concepts. Practical conversations about patients, the psychoanalysts believed, could help residents understand what it means to think psychodynamically more than conceptual work with abstract psychoanalytic concepts.[1] Unlike didactic lectures, case discussions positioned residents as active participants in the application of psychodynamic frames. But such participation did not come easy to the junior residents who, though used to the format of clinical case presentations and discussions, had only engaged in such exercises with a biopsychiatric frame. The psychodynamic approach confounded them. Initially, they engaged in these exercises reluctantly, and when they did so, the residents found their biopsychiatric tool kit ill suited to the task of projecting competence. These frictions activated the residents' skepticism, and they turned to expressions of doubt to assert a modicum of worth in this context.

JUNIOR RESIDENTS' INITIAL RELUCTANCE

Early in their training, the residents had yet to develop the skills necessary for being productive participants in psychodynamic conversations. This became evident during Terry's discussion with the residents who were in their second postgraduate year (PGY-2). Shortly before 8:00 a.m., Terry and I entered a brightly lit conference room at the hospital where the residents were working on the inpatient unit. We were greeted by a group of doctors wearing their white coats—an unusual sight for me, since their colleagues at the clinic went without them. A little more than three months away from finishing their inpatient rotations, the residents were now facing the prospect of shifting approaches. They were to begin meeting regularly with psychoanalytic supervisors and treating psychodynamic patients. This was Terry's first lecture to this cohort, and he was eager to start their doctoring overhaul. But the white coats, in addition to the conversation that ensued, underscored how far these PGY-2s were from the world of psychodynamic psychotherapy.

Terry began the two-hour lecture with a discussion of Stella, a patient he had treated in psychoanalysis years before. She had been referred to him by her "primary care doc," he explained, and had "had several months of feeling depressed, had been started on medication, and it only partially ameliorated the feelings." The psychiatric portion of his presentation dispatched with in mere seconds, Terry proceeded to describe Stella's upbringing, her relationships with her parents and theirs with each other, her history of intimate relationships, as well as the persistent relational troubles that had driven her to seek help. He made no mention of her symptoms or her medications, their dosages or effects.

As he moved into a description of treatment, Terry focused on Stella's experiences. He began with her "ambivalence about getting started. [. . .] She worked very hard, she felt, to resist doing certain things in the treatment that were normal, such as lying down on the couch to use for associations. Also, the billing practices were things that had to get worked out step by step." Further, Terry told the residents, "She [. . .] talked about feeling that she didn't want to succumb to an arbitrary authority, that being me." Terry went on to describe a traumatic hospitalization that Stella had suffered as a small child, her problems at work, and her dissatisfaction with two relationships and with her then-single state.

After completing the case presentation, Terry asked the residents whether "anything came to mind" about the material. The open-endedness of the question seemed to confound them; they were slow to respond. Three months into my fieldwork, I had come to recognize the question as an opening to begin hypothesizing about how Stella's behaviors in treatment and her relationship with Terry reflected her psychic difficulties. But the psychiatrists had not yet developed the acumen or knowledge required to engage in such psychodynamic thinking. They seemed ill at ease hypothesizing about Stella's inner life. Some took a chance, noting her troubles getting close in her intimate relationships yet being disappointed when they fell apart. At Terry's nudging, the residents turned their attention to the treatment itself:

Rashida (PGY-2): You did mention a couple of situations in which she became very uncomfortable in situations of conflict.
Terry (Instructor): What about those?
Rashida: The conversation about money, how to pay for the psychoanalysis, the meeting where she got upset about something that happened [at work], it suggests that she had difficulty with conflict.
Terry: What kind of difficulty?
Rashida: She was in a fog, she almost disassociates or something . . .
Terry: Uhm-hm! Does that ring any bells for you all? In this story?
[*Pause. No answer.*]

Terry: It's reminiscent of, it certainly brought to my mind, what a child experiences when a child is in [the hospital]. [*Terry goes on to remind the residents of Stella's hospitalization when she was a small child.*]

[*Pause. No further comments from the residents.*]

Terry: What about this whole idea about keeping things at bay, keeping things at a distance? Any thoughts about that? She's kept her relationships at bay, she's kept her work successes at bay. She worked hard in her early sessions to . . . in effect, to keep me at bay. What could be contributing? Dissociative is not a bad word to apply here.

Heather (PGY-2): Does it have something to do with it happening when she was most distressed? When she had [to go to the hospital] she was [. . .] kept in [a] fog [and] away from everybody.

Terry: So that, what you're positing, then, is that that may have gotten programmed with her as a way of responding to acute distress. So that got laid down.

[*Pause. No comments from the residents.*]

Terry: So these are all ideas about how this particular individual worked with her experiences.

The residents kept mostly quiet, reluctant to conjecture about Stella's difficulties in psychodynamic terms. Long pauses, interrupted by Terry's elaborations and encouragement, signaled their unfamiliarity with the task of a psychodynamic case discussion. Though they had participated in dozens of biopsychiatric case discussions, they found themselves on unfamiliar terrain in the psychodynamic version. Rashida (PGY-2) and Heather (PGY-2) hesitantly offered up hypotheses that, in their brevity and open-endedness, hinted at their own uncertainty. For his part, Terry did the lion's share of cognitive and interactional work in the exchange, helping the residents see the patient's troubles within the new framework. First, he edited and repackaged Stella's history and treatment to make it easier for the residents to connect the two. Next, during the conversation, he asked leading questions, seeking to draw the novices toward particular ideas and explanations. He picked up residents' specific words and offered positive feedback ("Dissociative is not a bad word to apply here."). When he heard a hint of insight from one of them, he amplified it, offering not only positive reinforcement but also implicit instruction in the kind of contributions that would be most valued in psychodynamic case discussions.

Such exercises were useful for exposing the residents to psychodynamic thinking, but they also revealed the friction inherent in their positions. Though these junior residents were relatively skilled psychiatrists, they were novice psychodynamic therapists. Unsure of what to say and how to say it, the residents retreated into silence. At this stage, Terry, Patricia, and the residents' supervisors played prominent roles guiding them toward a psychodynamic epistemic framework. But for such guidance to pay off, the residents would have to venture out of their initial reluctance and try out psychodynamic approaches themselves.

THE CHALLENGES OF THINKING PSYCHODYNAMICALLY EARLY IN TRAINING

When they arrived at the clinic, the residents became regular participants in the weekly meeting of the psychodynamic rotation. In this setting, they heard their more experienced colleagues and the occasional psychoanalyst deliver case presentations and participated in discussions about patients. These conversations were fertile ground for initiation into the psychodynamic epistemic culture. Early on, however, the residents were mired in epistemic friction.

This friction became evident during a case presentation by a junior resident. Jacob (PGY-3) was less than six months into his psychodynamic training but had agreed to present an ongoing treatment. Though senior residents were required to present cases as they neared graduation, for the junior residents this was only encouraged. Typically, the juniors would simply ask questions about psychodynamic treatments, forgoing the significant work of preparing and delivering a psychodynamic case presentation. But, in one of the few exceptions to this unspoken norm, Jacob had volunteered to present.

Jacob's difficulties and the friction he was confronting would soon become apparent. He began with an admission: "I wanna apologize 'cause my computer battery just died when I turned it on." When he suggested waiting until the following meeting or just presenting the case from memory, Terry opted for both. That day, Jacob would simply rely on his memory. It quickly became evident that, without his written notes, he just fell back on the epistemic frame in which he had already become competent, that of biological psychiatry.

He started by explaining that his patient, Chloe, had first seen him for medication management, but that they had transitioned into psychodynamic treatment after her previous therapist—another resident— graduated.[2] Jacob continued, "I've seen this patient maybe about thirty times.[3] She's had a history of Bipolar 1 and one hospitalization, and that hasn't been active since that time. Symptoms that have been active have been primarily anxiety, and occasionally she has depressive symptoms." Already, Jacob's presentation diverged from those I had seen his senior colleagues deliver. After describing some of Chloe's symptoms in greater detail, Jacob proceeded to explain that she is "pretty high functioning and has no trouble showing up for appointments on time and complying with medication regimes." He then gave a brief overview of the therapies Chloe had already undergone. Jacob then clarified: "My supervisor suggested that she could be a really good learning case, and I presented to her the option to begin psychodynamic therapy with me and she took that on immediately." At this point, Patricia interjected:

> Patricia (Instructor): Jacob, can I stop you, I have a question. What you gave was a traditional psychiatric presentation. . . . How would she introduce herself? If I walk up to her and presented myself, and I tell her my name, that I'm a psychologist and I have kids, [what would she say]?
>
> Jacob (PGY-3): She would identify herself as someone who's in a relationship, a hard worker, [who has] a lot of frequent anxiety which she doesn't really know where it comes from. . . . She checks under her bed, she worries about people who don't call . . . She also has some social anxiety as well. . . . She probably would say that she has some trouble interacting with people . . .
>
> Patricia: So this is how she introduced herself to you . . .
>
> Jacob: Right now, she's actually quite stable in the sense that I would be shocked if she showed up in PES [psychiatric emergency services], unlike a lot of my other patients . . .
>
> Patricia: Does she identify with her work?
>
> Jacob: She does computer-related work.

Jacob had a hard time stepping out of the psychiatric frame. Partly because of his prior training and partly because he continued to treat Chloe with medications, he could not set aside the typical psychiatric concerns with diagnoses and symptoms ("anxiety" and "depressive symptoms," a "history of Bipolar 1"), treatment history ("one hospitalization") and adherence ("complying with medication regimes"). Without the aid of his process notes, the resident simply fell back on the model of doctoring he had already internalized: that of biopsychiatry.

For her part, Patricia wanted to steer the residents toward understanding patients as people rather than as collections of symptoms and medical histories. She proposed a hypothetical scenario: how would Chloe introduce herself if, rather than meeting in a doctor's office, she had had a more informal encounter with Jacob? The imagined "conversation at a bar" was a favorite tool for psychoanalytic supervisors trying to teach vexed psychiatrists new ways of thinking about and talking with patients. Jacob nevertheless had a difficult time transitioning to this different epistemic frame: though he offered some bits of information about Chloe's life, he quickly returned to the manifestations of her disease and its trajectory.

Despite more than two dozen meetings with his patient—at least half of which were in psychodynamic treatment—Jacob had yet to develop the epistemic vision necessary to doctor in this approach. Instead, he remained tethered to biopsychiatry, leaving little room for attending to the patient's life, relationships, and feelings. Indeed, without process notes, Jacob could do little to obscure how deeply biopsychiatry had shaped his thinking. His case presentation epitomized the epistemic friction in the residents' roles. It also hinted at the professional struggles they confronted. Although the discussion would help Jacob along the path toward psychodynamic competence, it was not without the unease of critique. He was confronting again the challenges of novicehood but doing so from the position of an already trained professional. He knew how to deliver a "traditional psychiatric presentation" and how to help his patient manage her symptoms with medications. But this knowledge was insufficient, even misguided, in the psychodynamic rotation. Instead of a display of competence, Jacob's presentation only underscored the epistemic and professional contradictions he faced.

EXPRESSING AND MANAGING SKEPTICISM IN GROUP CONVERSATIONS

Skepticism was the inevitable corollary of such contradictions, and the less psychodynamically experienced residents turned to expressions of doubt to assert their worth. This was not yet the productive form of skepticism that can facilitate the acquisition of new knowledge. Instead, the junior residents approached psychodynamic assumptions as biopsychiatrists, outsiders critiquing an approach with which they were only beginning to gain some familiarity. At this point, the residents' skepticism was defensive, insulating them from the professional identity threats that came with learning how to doctor without drugs.

This became especially evident during a conversation in the psychodynamic rotation. When Terry introduced the trainees to the psychoanalytic concept of *resistance*, the impediments that patients put up to avoid doing something they unconsciously fear, he began with examples from his clinical work. One, which elicited the residents' laughter, entailed a patient who, "after a difficult session [. . .] calls and says, 'by the way, I'm going on vacation over the next four months, and I'm leaving tomorrow night.'" Some of the advanced residents shared their own experiences with patients' missed sessions, but Ely, a junior PGY-3, asked with a hint of frustration:

Ely (PGY-3): When is it dangerous to explore every red herring? Because I have some trouble thinking of every missed appointment as a resistance, whereas my [psychoanalytic] supervisor thinks that they are all

resistance. . . . Now I've come to believe that it is more resistance than
I originally thought, but . . . do I look for patterns? How can I tell when
it is resistance, and when the patient just has a legitimate reason to
miss session!?
Patricia (Instructor): Well, you have to look at the stage that you're at . . .
Terry (Instructor): Yes, that's a good question. . . . What is a cigar? It's a
cigar, but it can also be other things.

Ely packaged his doubts in ignorance: "Do I look for patterns? How
can I tell when it is resistance?" Yet it was clear that what he was expressing was not simply a novice's uncertainty but also a psychiatrist's
misgivings. Ely's question, I would later learn, was motivated by Nina,
a patient who, as Ely put it then, had "legitimate" reasons to miss her
therapy appointments. A successful professional, Nina took frequent trips
that led her to cancel sessions, sometimes at the last minute. Ely's doubts
about whether such "red herrings" were indeed "resistance" reflected
his biomedical training wherein he only needed to focus on a relatively
narrow set of indicators of disease rather than question every aspect of
patients' demeanor in treatment. Though he had "come to believe" that
there was "more resistance" than he had initially anticipated, he had yet
to adopt his supervisor's psychodynamic perspective, one in which Nina's
absences signaled her efforts at avoiding the intimacy of a therapeutic
relationship.[4]
More than illuminating Ely's doubts, the exchange also showcased how
his psychodynamic instructors and his more senior colleagues engaged
with his skeptical questioning. Terry and Patricia did not dismiss the junior resident's comments as novice ignorance. They might have easily
done so that day: Ely's was the lone voice of doubt during the conversation. Instead, they offered practical advice ("look at the stage") and
validation ("that's a good question"). These actions could reinforce the
psychodynamic perspective without dismissing the resident's skepticism
or the friction he was confronting. For their part, senior residents showcased their own facility with the psychodynamic frame. Whether a patient
canceled a session after the resident had to miss one, took a vacation
abruptly after a resident's own, or called, as Zoli (PGY-4) shared, "half
an hour before a session to tell me that he was in New York," Ely's more
experienced colleagues amplified their instructors' view. These residents
engaged in the discussion from a psychodynamic rather than a biopsychiatric perspective. Ely, earlier in the process, could not yet channel a similar
epistemic generosity. Yet his doctoring overhaul was already under way
in these collective settings.

Developing Self-Reflexivity on the Path to Competence

The residents found the psychodynamic mandate that they attend to the dynamics of their relationships with patients dissonant and challenging. In biopsychiatry, they received little explicit instruction in the nuances of such relationships. Beyond communicating empathy, managing professional boundaries, and attending to safety concerns, the residents had given their interactions with patients little thought. Pharmacological work did not seem to require it. In contrast, psychodynamic treatments require clinicians to tune into the affective undercurrents of their relationships with patients and do so by paying close attention to their own emotions.[5] In this approach, the residents must widen their analytic lens to include not just their patients' inner lives but also their own. The following pages show them first coming to terms with their new doctoring roles and then beginning to reflect and work on themselves to better inhabit such roles. Cultivating self-reflexivity is, in turn, an essential step toward psychodynamic competence.

RECOGNIZING AND COMING TO TERMS WITH PSYCHODYNAMIC DOCTORING

The contours of psychodynamic doctoring roles came into focus slowly, over many conversations about working with patients. But one such discussion, prompted by a psychoanalyst's case presentation, was especially productive in this respect. It revealed the stark contrasts between the residents' existing doctoring assumptions and those they would need to accommodate themselves to in psychodynamic psychotherapy. The junior residents, preoccupied with epistemic and professional frictions, met the psychoanalyst's focus on the interactional dynamics of a session and their affective significance with skepticism. Nevertheless, the discussion was just the catalyst they needed to recognize what psychodynamic doctoring would require of them. Though uncomfortable, this knowledge was essential for their self-reflexivity and, eventually, competence in this approach.

Ted, an experienced psychoanalyst who also served as a supervisor for some of the residents in the program, had visited the psychodynamic rotation several times to discuss an ongoing treatment. His patient, Sophia, suffered from long-term depression associated with a host of interpersonal problems. That day, Ted began with a typical psychodynamic case presentation: he reminded the residents about Sophia's relational troubles and proceeded to read process notes of a recent session. The discussion that followed focused partly on Sophia and partly on the therapist himself.

One exchange from the session captured the residents' interest. As Ted described it, Sophia had had a Freudian slip in the session—saying "scream saver" rather than "screen saver" to refer to the family photos she had put on her computer screen.[6] The patient, partly embarrassed, wondered aloud what the slip might have meant. In typical psychoanalytic fashion, Ted followed Sophia's lead and asked what she made of the notion of "saving screams." As they explored the theme, the patient slowly revealed her feelings toward her therapist: how little she still trusted him months into treatment and how she had continued to withhold key parts of herself from him. The residents recognized their own struggles in those of the experienced psychoanalyst. But, in dealing with this common challenge, Ted had adopted a strategy that diverged from what the residents would have done:

> Andrea (PGY-3): I thought it was interesting that you kind of kept the material right where she was that day, talking about how if she let out her grief in your office that it might be too loud. . . . And this is probably my, you know, the fact that I'm still new at this, that I would have taken everything and tried to make it more of a global sort of overall, how does it fit into these things that you're kind of [worried about]. So I thought that it was interesting that you stayed right where she was.
>
> Terry (Instructor): Why . . . and I don't think what you're saying is . . . a lot of that . . . that's how a lot of therapists feel about that kind of stuff. But anybody have thoughts as to why a therapist would wanna take a specific statement and make it global?
>
> Lucas (PGY-3): I think there are a lot of reasons!
>
> Terry: Well?
>
> Lucas: One of them would be that it's, there's more tension in keeping things in the here and now! I mean, it's a lot harder for a patient and sometimes therapist to look at feelings about you in the moment and it becomes much more personal, and intimate and close [. . .]. The other thing that also, at least that's been true for me that I, I tend to not appreciate that therapy is another relationship that the patient has. . . . So I feel, I'm always looking . . . you know, how does this connect with your chief complaint, or what you came in with [. . .]. It took me a while, I guess, to realize that these things are all happening at the same time, and so while it is, yes, also about the concrete manifest content, it's also often a message to me that gets played out.

Ted's approach proved puzzling to the residents: there was nothing obvious about his strategy to, as Andrea put it, "stay right where [the patient] was" in the session. Zaheed (PGY-3), another junior resident, confessed that he would have viewed Sophia's comment as "just a slip" and moved on. But the residents were realizing that it was precisely by attending to the patient's moment-by-moment utterances and feelings that Ted was able to better understand her continued reluctance to disclose more of herself to him. For the junior psychiatrists, adopting a similar strategy would require shifting their thinking away from the medical frame that centered on patients' "global" concerns and their diagnoses, and focusing instead on their particular words and demeanor in session.

Such a focus was challenging on more than a cognitive level. It also required the residents to develop a new understanding of their roles and their relationships with patients. Lucas (PGY-3) articulated the residents' predicament later in the same exchange:

> I mean, in no other field of medicine and no other place within the field of psychiatry [are you] really supposed to look at yourself as being particularly important because the patient has [you as] a relational object, as opposed to a service provider and somebody with a fiduciary obligation towards that person. So it really is a whole different way of thinking. [. . .]. I mean, people are even afraid to write in the first pronoun in notes! You'll see "this clinician," "this author," "this writer"! It's like *I* should be somehow out of the picture. So it's just a very different way of thinking! You know, that this is about in some ways you personally and this space right here, right now.

Lucas's colleagues knew that he was not simply responding to Ted's presentation but was also speaking from experience: he, too, was treating a patient whose contradictory feelings toward him had become evident during sessions. Yet his earlier training had not prepared him to think about what was happening at these moments in the relationship. Instead, along with his colleagues, he had to navigate several epistemic and role contradictions: between thinking of patients' "chief complaint" and their "feelings about you in the moment," between being "a service provider" with a "fiduciary obligation towards" the patient and being a patient's "relational object," between thinking of themselves in the third person ("'this clinician,' 'this author,' 'this writer'") and the first person ("*I* should be somehow out of the picture").[7] How might "this clinician" manage the conundrums of psychodynamic relationships in which interactions "right here, right now," as Lucas put it, are "more personal, and intimate and close"? "A year and a half ago," Lucas continued, the residents would have thought that it was "extremely . . . unempathic and rude" to focus on the treatment relationship and discuss—*with patients*—how they felt about it. During their psychiatric training, they had learned that their mandate was to attend to patients' primary concerns as evidenced by their symptoms. Connecting such concerns with the relationship was not part of their field of vision.

In contrast, psychodynamic psychotherapy offered the residents a different view of caring for their patients. For Lucas, this even prompted a reassessment of a typical pharmacologic appointment. "The patient," he explained, "might experience" a superficial expression of empathy during a discussion of their "chief complaint" as "essentially neglecting them, because we're not bringing in the here and now, which is where they're experiencing their feeling." A more caring stance, inspired by psychodynamic technique, would have the residents attend to patients' moment-by-moment expressions so as to better understand them and their feelings. This would require that the residents reimagine their doctoring roles and their practical work.

Lucas's comments revealed the awareness and self-reflexivity necessary for developing a growing facility with psychodynamic practices. About two-thirds of the way through the third postgraduate year, Lucas was increasingly able to articulate the gaps and contradictions between his biopsychiatric training and what he was learning in the psychodynamic rotation. In turn, acknowledging and discussing these sources of friction in the group could help him and his colleagues along the path to competence. After all, Lucas could not speak with his patient about the challenges he faced—in sessions, he had to inhabit the role of psychodynamic therapist, as incongruous as it may have felt. And while he could talk with his psychoanalytic supervisor, the supervisor's advice did not resonate in the same way as his peers' affirmation. Lucas was not the only one who would have missed the significance of Sophia's "scream saver"—his colleagues admitted to a similar oversight. In each other's company, the residents could be remarkably honest about the contradictions between being pharmacologists and being psychodynamic psychotherapists. In the group, they could also hone the self-reflexivity necessary to shift their doctoring practices away from a singular focus on psychiatric doctoring and toward greater acceptance of psychodynamic roles.

EXPERIMENTING WITH SELF-REFLEXIVITY

Terry and Patricia actively encouraged the residents' self-reflexivity by orienting group discussions toward the patient *and* the therapist. A resident delivering a case presentation would thus expect questions and comments not only about their patient and the treatment but also about themselves and their actions. Though uncomfortable, such inquiries facilitated self-awareness and self-work, allowing the residents—presenter and audience alike—to experiment with psychodynamic doctoring roles.

A week after Jacob's (PGY-3) computer mishap, the resident returned with printed copies of his process notes. This time, the presentation would take a different course. Jacob began with a brief introduction that interwove biopsychiatric and psychodynamic concerns:

> The patient that I'm presenting had been seeing me for about two to three months of weekly therapy, had a history of bipolar disorder, and had one episode of mania, has ongoing issues with anxiety, and had just ended a long relationship that had been ambivalent. . . . She had been coping over the last couple of sessions with the idea of being single, and meeting different people . . .

Though he still led with the patient's diagnosis and symptoms, Jacob was beginning to shift his frame of reference by describing Chloe's interpersonal troubles. He proceeded to read from his process notes. He explained that he had scheduled the psychodynamic session "at 5:00 p.m., and there was some misunderstanding with the front desk about whether [Chloe] was really scheduled to come in or whether that was a mistake." Recall from chapter 2 that the residents had little flexibility to create time for psychodynamic appointments in their schedule. Some, Jacob included, chose to extend their work hours for that purpose. His efforts at managing these temporal constraints caused more than bureaucratic consternation. When Chloe "did show up," Jacob continued, "[the front desk] called me to confirm that we had an appointment, and this was all happening with her standing right there." Jacob thus began their interaction in the lobby by apologizing to his patient "about the confusion at the desk," an apology that, the resident pointed out, Chloe met with a small laugh. In describing such details, Jacob was beginning to showcase his understanding of the broader domain of interactions he had to attend to in psychodynamic psychotherapy.

"When we got into the office," Jacob continued, "I asked [Chloe] how her week went, and she said that 'there were some good things, some not so good things, and some neutral things.'" He paused and then explained to the group: "A quick comment on that: two or three sessions ago, to get things going [in the session] I said, 'are there some good things that had happened and some not so good things?' Later, when I presented my process notes [to my supervisor], I realized that that had become a pattern." Though still struggling to act psychodynamically in sessions—struggles that his process notes laid bare—Jacob was demonstrating a growing awareness of his doctoring practices through his case presentation.

As the session started, Chloe "was beaming, because she had a date for the night." The patient, Jacob explained, had difficult relationships with men, including her father, a theme that had become increasingly central in the treatment. During their meeting, upon learning the news of her upcoming date, the resident offered an encouraging "That's great!" For the next several minutes in his presentation, Jacob continued to read through his notes of the session, giving a word-by-word account of a conversation that centered on Chloe's challenges breaking off an earlier relationship. To my ears, the resident had shown that he could do something other than pharmacology: he could talk with Chloe about her life and delve deeper into her emotional and relational troubles.

But in the discussion that followed, it became evident that the case presentation, though better crafted than that of the previous week, had not fully succeeded in establishing Jacob's psychodynamic competence. Though he had done a better job of inhabiting a psychodynamic role in the presentation, Terry made clear that Jacob had done less well in the session. To my surprise, Jacob's encouraging response to Chloe's upcoming date garnered critique. Terry began:

> One way to think about that is as a reflection in the transference and countertransference [. . .]. Somehow, in the room with this patient, is that things are primed in such a way that she says something and you say "that's great." [. . .] As a therapist you can say that you're reflecting her positive feelings and that's being empathic, and that's quite true. On the other hand, it sets up a system between the two where the patient is conditioned over time to only bring in the things that she's getting positive feedback for, and not bring in things that will make the treater sad. You'd be amazed at what patients recall and how they feel its effect.

Though couched in psychoanalytic language, Terry's point was clear: Jacob's attempt at being supportive was actually psychodynamically counterproductive. Already primed to mimic her therapist's language, Chloe could, unconsciously, become "conditioned over time to only bring in the things that she's getting positive feedback for." This, in turn, could cement her resistance toward uncovering more troubling experiences. Patient and therapist were inadvertently colluding in closing off avenues toward unearthing her less positive, and also less conscious, feelings. Still, akin to the previous week, Terry identified the problem in Jacob's attempt at psychodynamic doctoring all the while remaining supportive of the resident.

He invited the group to reflect on Jacob's performance. The resident's more experienced colleagues readily chimed in. Carson (PGY-4) offered less prescriptive ways to respond to the patient's disclosure: "You could say, 'Wow, you seem really happy!' or 'Wow, you're beaming!'" Lucas, now a wiser PGY-4, explained, showcasing his own self-awareness, "I think in the room about my mind and [the patient's] mind, and then I try to think about things about whether they're on my or their mind." In Jacob's case, "that's great" was on his, rather than Chloe's mind. With patients, Lucas clarified, this meant making observations that are "very clear that this is what I think I heard." Over time, the resident explained, "I get more and more careful about what I let come from me." Jacob was letting too much of his "mind" show in "the room," to borrow Lucas's formulation. He had yet to inhabit the kind of interactional restraint characteristic of doctoring psychodynamically. For his part, Lucas was acting as a surrogate instructor, framing Jacob's misstep in psychodynamic terms, while also demonstrating his own competence in the approach.

To be sure, self-reflexivity was not only the domain of advanced residents. Jacob had already signaled his advances on this front when he identified the interactional pattern that had come to dominate his sessions with Chloe. Later, he shared with his colleagues, "One thing I noticed is that sometimes I have difficulty separating between a CBT psycho-education approach and a psychodynamic approach." Training in both therapies simultaneously, Jacob was having trouble keeping them apart in his work with Chloe. "So I try to jump in there and identify distortions," Jacob explained, using a term typically used in CBT to describe patients' unrealistic thoughts. "That can be seen as I'm a fixer," he stressed, choosing a word that was meaningful to his patient. Chloe had described her own father as a "fixer," and Jacob was becoming cognizant of the fact that he was increasingly occupying that same role. "One thing that I've talked to my supervisor about was that I need to make sure to give her space to bring in new issues and problems," Jacob explained.

The resident needed to shift his conversational patterns away from the more directive style common in CBT and pharmacology and more toward the open-endedness typical in the psychodynamic approach. With the aid of process notes and conversations with his supervisor and his colleagues, he could identify and reflect on this doctoring conundrum. But, in revealing his mistake, Jacob did more than acknowledge the challenges of transitioning from one way of doctoring to another. He also demonstrated his growing awareness of how his interactional choices affected the dynamics of the therapeutic relationship. Though he could not yet successfully inhabit a psychodynamic doctoring role with his patient, Jacob could, in the company of his mentors and peers, exhibit a growing understanding of what stood in the way.

This and other such discussions were illuminating on two counts. First, they revealed the contrasting epistemic machineries the residents had to inhabit. Second, they also showcased the roles that supervisors, instructors, and colleagues played in fostering junior residents' psychodynamic competence. With their supervisors, the residents could examine their existing doctoring approach and work toward improvement. For their part, Terry and Patricia made self-reflection an explicit part of the training, regularly inviting trainees to unpack their own, their colleagues', or, at times, invited psychoanalysts' doctoring performances. And, as the residents advanced in their training, they progressed from being uneasy objects of such analysis to becoming competent agents of it. With time, their psychodynamic doctoring performances showcased their competence and amounted to veritable professional testimonials.

Offering Professional Testimonials and Managing Skepticism Collectively

Toward the end of their residencies, psychiatrists in the fourth postgraduate year routinely delivered case presentations in the psychodynamic meetings. More than rituals marking the completion of the residents' training in this approach, these presentations had dual functions. On a basic level, they delineated the contours of psychodynamic treatments and clarified their stakes for the junior residents. Unlike in pharmacology or CBT, where symptom improvement was a key marker of a treatment's success, in psychodynamic therapy patients' insights into the roots of their problems were deemed more important for their betterment. Additionally, senior residents' case presentations served to reassure their more skeptical junior colleagues. While psychoanalytic supervisors and instructors could affirm that a patient benefited from treatment, hearing colleagues themselves describe patients' and their own deeper self-understanding or insight carried greater weight. Such professional testimonials were essential conduits for the collective management of skepticism.

SEEING AND SHARING CHANGES IN PATIENTS AND THEMSELVES

Akin to CBT, the residents' psychodynamic competence did not depend on cure. Yet here, unlike in the more pragmatic cognitive and behavioral approaches, they had few practical hooks for displaying their abilities. There were no behavioral modification or thought exercises they could implement successfully in role-plays or with their patients. Instead, sharing psychodynamic successes revolved around constructing particular narratives about patients, the treatment, and themselves. Repeatedly, experienced residents delivered case presentations that followed similar scripts: they began with descriptions of early challenges around patients' disclosure, session attendance, or trust; then moved to the residents' renewed commitment to building the treatment relationship; and ended with the payoffs for both patient and resident. In this framework, sustained psychodynamic work resulted in eventual successes at fostering patients' insight and residents' own new competencies.[8]

Toward the end of his residency, Ely, now an experienced senior resident, delivered a lengthy case presentation about his work with Nina. Whereas earlier in the program he had doubted his psychodynamic supervisor's and instructors' observations, he had come to adopt a similar lens for understanding her treatment behaviors. Nina's absences had persisted throughout their work together and, as Ely contemplated graduation, he brought up the treatment's trajectory to his patient. He explained to the group that they "had [recently] missed quite a few sessions," but, with his departure mere weeks away, Ely wanted to have "a big talk about where are we going from here." His supervisor, Ely explained, had been "pushing all along" for more "regular" sessions, and the resident finally followed through on that advice. He offered Nina the option to either stop therapy altogether or to continue with a more "regular" schedule.

Ely explained to his colleagues that, in the session, he placed Nina's decision in psychodynamic terms, connecting her treatment absences with her relational patterns. The resident read from his process notes what he had told his patient: "I'm wondering if that's how other people feel in relationships with you, if you stay on the surface and things just kind of drift apart." Ely had managed to place Nina's lack of commitment to treatment—as evidenced by her absences and her general resistance to talking about herself—in the context of her broader troubles with intimacy. Though she did not commit to that explanation "in the moment," Nina returned "the next session [and] said 'I thought about what we talked about last time.'"

Taking a break from reading his process notes, Ely told his colleagues, "That's huge for her." The intervention had paid off: Nina committed to meeting "through June," the point when Ely would graduate. As they began meeting "regularly," she showed a newfound openness to self-examination. Ely also "noticed a change in myself": whereas he was "somewhat dreading going in," and "felt like [he] was doing more work than she was," after this discussion "things got easier." Ely shared, "I found myself enjoying going in and looking forward to seeing her." Significantly, "the supervision got easier." Inhabiting the same epistemic framework as his supervisor allowed the resident to better navigate the conundrums of that relationship and those of the psychodynamic treatment.

And while Ely had already established the utility of the psychodynamic approach in fostering some self-knowledge for his patient, the rest of his presentation revealed that his work was not done. But now, Ely needed no prodding to doctor psychodynamically. After having had a few good sessions with his patient, the tide was once again turning.

> *Ely (PGY-4)*: We talked about ending and I asked if she had any thoughts about that. And I wanted to pick an end date, and I thought that that may actually make it more real for her, and we actually picked an end date. And I asked, "How do you feel about leaving?" and, in her classic style, she shrugged and said, "I think I'll be OK." My temptation is to say, "We've seen each other a year, and saw each other for so many hours, what do you mean you don't care?!"
>
> [*Much laughter around the room as Ely's annoyance is evident.*]
>
> *Terry (Instructor)* [*jokingly echoing Ely's tone*]: What am I, chopped liver?
>
> [*Continued laughter.*]
>
> *Ely*: Well, that's how I felt! But I feel like this is something that I want to bring up.

Ely no longer needed to seek advice from his supervisor about how to proceed. He already knew that Nina's response and his own reaction were something "to bring up" in their next session. Deploying a psychodynamic perspective, he identified Nina's "resistance" and the links between the therapeutic relationship and her interpersonal troubles. He also showcased his self-reflexivity, making his frustration evident to the group, his feelings fodder for the analytic mill. In turn, this prompted Terry's validation, as he amplified Ely's feelings ("What am I, chopped liver?"), affirming their importance for the treatment. Edward, an experienced psychoanalyst who had come to the meeting to comment on Ely's presentation, offered further endorsement: "Neurotic people make you feel parental, and character-ological people make you feel like they feel. I think there's some charac-terological stuff at work there, so I think you're on the right track." These remarks once again made clear that Ely had successfully transitioned from the skeptical junior resident to the competent senior resident who could ably doctor psychodynamically.

Ely's presentation was compelling testimony to the utility of the psycho-dynamic approach. Though his patient's relational troubles remained, Ely had helped her better understand what caused them. He also had come to experience doctoring in a new way. But it had taken more than Ely's work with Nina to convince him that her actions (or, rather, inactions) were a form of "resistance" that epitomized her "difficulties" with building close relationships. Shifting his epistemic framework depended on two years' worth of weekly meetings with his psychoanalytic supervisor and with col-leagues and instructors in the psychodynamic group. His case presentation was testimony to the effects of such immersion on Ely's earlier skepticism.

No longer the doubting biopsychiatrist, Ely was now the psychodynamic initiate who could affirm the utility of the approach.

Ely's experience was far from unique. A year earlier, Kai had shared with his colleagues his own trajectory from skepticism to competence. When Kai (PGY-4) presented his work with Carl, a patient who had had trouble opening up during the treatment, he made clear that, early in the training, he had harbored significant doubts about whether a psychodynamic approach was possible. Kai explained that his "patient was very concrete and thought and talked about, mostly about medical issues." The resident clarified, "Rarely did Carl talk about his feelings, other than to say that he would cut people off on the road if he was angry." In his third postgraduate year at that point, Kai was skeptical of a psychodynamic treatment, and he turned to his psychoanalytic supervisor for advice. His supervisor encouraged the resident to remain committed to the treatment and to begin paying more attention to his own feelings.

As Kai (PGY-4) continued with the presentation, he painted a picture of his patient's progress and, in turn, of his own diminishing doubts. With time, Carl had begun sharing more about his day-to-day life and struggles, moving away from an exclusive focus on somatic concerns. He became more attuned to and open about his inner life. Kai too started to feel more "comfortable" in sessions. He told his colleagues that he felt Carl had made a great deal of progress and shared process notes that lent credence to his conviction.

But, with Kai's graduation, treatment was nearing its inevitable end, giving rise to new challenges. The resident reflected, "Part of my countertransference is that I feel really good that he's getting better, but I feel impatient that things are getting good not as fast as I want." Kai's doubts had been supplanted by psychodynamic competence. As before, Kai relied on his supervisor for advice:

So it took me a while and talking to my supervisor [. . .] to really get a sense of what's getting in the way of talking further about this termination. And part of the reason it's him and part of the reason it's me, too, in that I was very cautious, and I didn't really want to feel that important because I [feel some] responsibility. So [my supervisor] kind of convinced me over the weeks that this guy has worked well in sessions because he really trusts me, and he thinks . . . There's a lot of positive transference, and things have worked because I'm important, so when I'm leaving, that's gonna introduce a lot of issues, and I need to be aware that I do play a huge part in this guy's life. He never missed an appointment, basically.

Kai had come to accept an unusual professional role: "I do play a huge part in this guy's life." Carl had made this evident by "never miss[ing] an appointment," a behavior that psychotherapists frequently take as a sign of success. This was not the empathetic but relatively detached doctor-patient relationship Kai and his colleagues had come to expect in biopsychiatry. It was instead an intimate relationship that had developed over more than a year and that had resulted in changes in patient *and* clinician. Yet Kai felt uneasy. His "countertransference," as he technically described his emotions—namely, his hesitation about feeling "that important" and his guilt at "leaving" the patient just as he had started to show progress—had delayed more difficult and affectively nuanced conversations with Carl. For Kai, the necessity of working through these conundrums was self-evident. No longer the doubtful psychiatrist, he was a dedicated psychodynamic therapist.

Kai's presentation made for compelling testimony to the utility of a psychodynamic approach. Carl had arrived at the clinic deeply depressed and increasingly isolated but, after dozens of meetings with Kai, he was starting to face his unhappiness and express himself and his feelings. That the patient found the treatment productive was clear in his regular attendance and, as Kai explained, in his desire to attend his graduation. Kai too had become better attuned not only to his patient's inner life but also to his own. He had taken on a new doctoring role and was implicitly offering professional testimony to its benefits.

Terry and Patricia amplified Kai's implicit message. After thanking him, Patricia reflected that "termination is the hardest part," validating the resident's struggles and placing them in a psychodynamic framework. Terry commended Kai for the "wonderful material" he had presented, concluding, "This is really . . . wow!" Words eluded the typically eloquent psychoanalyst, but they were, in some sense, superfluous. Kai had delivered an exemplary performance of psychodynamic competence by showing himself to be an astute observer of his patient's emotional and relational troubles and a mindful participant in the therapeutic relationship. He adeptly deployed psychoanalytic language and revealed enough of himself to demonstrate the kind of self-reflexivity deemed necessary in psychodynamic work. The instructors' praise deepened the subtle but essential work Kai had done in the service of collectively managing skepticism.

Kai's presentation, with its emphasis on his own doubts and struggles, opened avenues for other residents to share their struggles with doctoring psychodynamically. It also showed them that competence was possible, if only with a sustained commitment to engaging with the approach not as observers but as participants. Finally, Kai's presentation affirmed that psychodynamic psychotherapy did indeed help patients, though in ways that diverged from other approaches. Recognizing such successes in their colleagues' descriptions of patients' (and sometimes their own) deepening self-knowledge did not always come easy for the residents. It was, nevertheless, an important stepping stone toward accepting psychodynamic interventions as legitimate alternatives to CBT and pharmacology.

MAKING PROFESSIONAL TESTIMONIES MORE COMPELLING BY ENROLLING PATIENTS

Few things helped in building such recognition than testimony from patients themselves, even when communicated indirectly. Leah's experience offered just such an opening toward bringing patients' own perspectives to the residents. A senior resident nearing graduation, Leah began the discussion by making clear that the treatment had had its share of struggles: her patient had arrived at their first session thirty minutes late, hostile to the task at hand—namely, talking with her. He continued to sporadically miss sessions throughout the treatment. Early on, he spent much of their time together describing his romantic conquests. But, despite such seeming barriers to self-reflection, and the temporal constraints the residents faced, Leah resolved to follow her supervisor's encouragement and meet with her patient three times a week.

To her surprise, she found the higher frequency of sessions productive. She shared with her colleagues that she had "liked" working so intensively. Though they had started treatment by meeting twice a week, when she and her patient committed to the additional session, "the relationship got closer" and they "had more things to talk about." When they "had to cut back to twice a week" because of the patient's schedule, Leah could sense a "distance between [them]," one that seemed to vanish as they returned to their more intensive rhythm. "I thought with three times a week we're gonna run out of things to talk about," Leah admitted, but, she declared, "it was the opposite." The patient opened up about his struggles with intimacy and his deep desire for it, and about a past abuse he had suffered at the hands of a caretaker. His openness then enabled insights into his relationships as an adult.

Though he continued to suffer from depression, as they approached the end of their treatment, the patient showed Leah that he had nevertheless benefited from their work together. Leah shared with her colleagues:

> So closer to the time of termination, one day he talked about not wanting to move on to another therapist, telling me that "you've been helpful." It was very moving, he was crying, and I almost felt like crying, and he said, "I just want you to know that you really made a difference," and he said that "wherever I move, I hope you have contacts there, because I would want to see someone that you recommend." He brought me a thank-you card, and I still have it actually!

Though the treatment had gotten off to a rocky start, Leah's commitment to working with her patient in a psychodynamic framework eroded his earlier reluctance, which, in turn, led to deeper connection and insight. Nevertheless, for the patient, work remained to be done. The situation was not unusual: the residents frequently found themselves in situations of having to end a treatment only to pass the patient on to another resident who was at an earlier stage in the program. But, as Barry, an experienced psychoanalyst in attendance for Leah's presentation, put it, the therapy had been sufficiently impactful: "[The patient] left treatment telling you that it is not all complete, and, my God, I'm a different person!" This validation, along with the patient's own words, served as compelling testimony to Leah's own shift from skeptical biopsychiatrist to competent psychodynamic initiate.

In addition, Leah's professional testimonial about the utility of the psychodynamic approach was made more compelling by the patient's own emotions and gratitude as their treatment came to an end. Such case presentations were thus more than simply opportunities for the residents to showcase their newfound competence. They were also powerful contributions to the collective management of skepticism, especially when patients' voices became part of the narrative. When Kai shared with his colleagues his patient's wish to come to his graduation, and Leah described her patient's heartfelt thanks, they were affirming that psychodynamic treatments worked. For earlier residents who struggled with the psychodynamic doctoring mandate, such professional testimonials were windows into new epistemic and professional possibilities.

Conclusion

Coming to psychodynamic training after years spent learning biomedicine, the residents were confronted with the realities of learning to doctor without drugs. Whether this meant presenting cases in new ways or reframing their understanding of patients' problems and their betterment, the residents found themselves on unstable terrain. And while much of their training focused on "learning by doing," treating patients was insufficient for developing new doctoring repertoires and navigating the frictions inherent in the process. With patients, the residents might feel their inexperience acutely or see their growing competence pay off, but they could not place their conundrums or successes within a psychodynamic framework.

Conversations with supervisors, instructors, and peers were best suited for facilitating the residents' transition from skepticism to psychodynamic competence. On the one hand, these discussions were generative of the kind of epistemically specific repertoires of action necessary for the residents to understand how to do psychodynamic psychotherapy. In these settings, the residents could learn how to talk to a patient *and* how to talk about them psychodynamically. On the other hand, group meetings offered the residents opportunities to express doubts, receive affirmation from instructors and peers, and witness colleagues engage with psychodynamic doctoring even as they had, months before, been doubtful of it. Group discussions were thus ideal sites for the residents to learn about the psychodynamic epistemic machinery while also recognizing and managing the ongoing struggles inherent in becoming participants in it.

Case presentations and discussions—the main form that such conversations took—have long garnered the attention of social scientists studying medical education. They reveal "how medicine constructs its objects," to quote anthropologist Byron Good, and are opportunities for the residents to engage in what organizational scholars have described as "sensemaking."[9] Sensemaking requires social actors to step back from "immersion in projects" to a more reflective stance oriented toward creating order out of action that had become "unintelligible in some way."[10] For the residents, puzzled by psychodynamic assumptions and skeptical of the intervention, being able to reflect on their conundrums in the company of peers and instructors was a key part of learning how to doctor in this approach.

Case presentations are also "exercises in self-presentation," as sociologist Renee Anspach has argued, illuminating the contours of competence in medicine.[11] These collective exercises—commonplace in medical training regardless of specialty—make clear that gaining competence is more than a growing facility with particular techniques and assumptions. It is also about successfully navigating the relationships that constitute a particular professional group.[12] Collective discussions of patients and treatments thus played an essential role in reshaping the residents' understandings of their doctoring roles and of themselves. Indeed, social scientists have long argued that identities are the emergent effects of interactions among social actors and are thus amenable to change.[13] New identities, sociologist Andreas Glaeser has proposed, become "compelling through the mutually supporting work of resonances, recognitions, and corroborations" constituted in relationships.[14] At Shorewood, group meetings offered residents opportunities for just such relational immersion and affirmation.

Instructors and supervisors were important interlocutors in the residents' search for epistemic grounding, offering corrections or praise in response to their case presentations and discussions. Their feedback was also significant in shaping the psychiatrists' expectations about the contours of psychodynamic competence. Yet it was peers' own contributions to such group conversations that made possible the work of reframing residents' doctoring roles and that of collectively managing skepticism.

As the residents tried to make sense of the disjunctures between what they expected doctoring to be and what they heard from their psychodynamic supervisors and instructors, they turned to one another for assurance. In the company of colleagues, residents could share bewilderment or skepticism at mentors' advice and question the very possibility of psychodynamic treatment when patients seemed unequal to the task. They could see that their struggles were not unique but also, and just as important, that they could be overcome. Put another way, colleagues could offer both validation and testimony about the possibilities of psychodynamic doctoring, facilitating the shift from skepticism to competence.

7 ∗ Competence and Resolution

Toward the end of their training, the residents' skepticism dwindles, giving way to psychotherapeutic competence. This, in turn, enables them to find resolutions to the frictions embedded in their roles. About two months into the rotation on cognitive behavioral therapy (CBT) for depression, Aaron, a resident in his third postgraduate year (PGY-3), offered a glimpse of what this might look like with a patient. The patient had come to the clinic seeking help with his anger outbursts. Though he was given a diagnosis of major depression, the patient insisted to Aaron during their appointment that he did not "want any medication" for his symptoms. Instead, the resident explained, "the whole session focused on how he can recognize his emotions better before he starts getting angry." For this, Aaron turned to CBT, "doing a thought record" and helping his patient identify unrealistic thinking while coming up with alternative thoughts. With little use for his core expertise in pharmacology, Aaron turned to CBT to successfully perform his doctoring role. He needn't have done so had his patient accepted a medication prescription. But Aaron was able to still offer care and enact his mandate with the use of his CBT tool kit. And, in telling his instructor and colleagues about this conundrum and his success in navigating it, the resident showcased his competence and offered testimony about CBT's usefulness. He also implicitly hinted at how he integrated the competing repertoires of pharmacology and psychotherapy: the former was his primary line of intervention, but when it did not offer a ready solution to a patient's problems, the latter filled in any remaining gaps.

The previous two chapters showed the residents learning to doctor psychotherapeutically and engage in the collective management of skepticism in the CBT (chapter 5) and psychodynamic (chapter 6) rotations. This chapter focuses on the residents' psychotherapeutic training as it nears its conclusion. No longer skeptical outsiders, the residents engage with psychotherapy on its own terms, showcasing their skills in doctoring performances that ably reflect the assumptions and practices of each therapeutic approach. The residents find that the professional frictions in their roles attenuate, if not entirely disappear, as they become increasingly confident and self-directed psychotherapy initiates. Competence also helps mitigate the epistemic friction with which the residents struggle. Some, akin to Aaron, move toward what I came to think of as pragmatic accommodation, remaining anchored in biopsychiatry but making use of psychotherapeutic interventions, typically cognitive and behavioral, as needed. A smaller number of residents demonstrate a deeper commitment to psychotherapy, usually psychodynamic, seeking to account for the biological *and* the relational dimensions of patients' problems. These doctors integrate biopsychiatric and psychodynamic epistemes, developing what I describe as hybrid repertoires.

The following pages reveal the residents' facility with CBT and psychodynamic skills, as well as the resolution of the contradictions with which they struggled. The first part of the chapter details the residents' performances of competence and their confidence in their psychotherapeutic roles. In CBT, I show them ably thinking through the nuances of patients' troubles and engaging in compelling role-plays. I also return to Sonora, the resident whose troubles I briefly discussed in chapter 3, and show her competently navigating her ongoing treatment conundrums. In psychodynamic psychotherapy, I offer an extended discussion of one resident's display of competence. Jake, a senior resident (PGY-4), delivered a case presentation complete with process notes that revealed his skills in constructing a psychodynamic narrative about the treatment relationship and conducting himself with sensitivity and attention in sessions. During the case discussion that followed, Jake showcased a nuanced analysis of his patient and of himself. The latter part of the chapter focuses on the residents' distinct approaches to epistemic resolution. I begin with pragmatic accommodation, the most common model, and show the residents deploying biopsychiatric and psychotherapeutic, typically CBT, interventions as needed. The chapter's final section turns to the residents who develop hybrid repertoires and reveals their strategies for integrating approaches as they seek to better understand and help their patients.

Performing Competence and Mitigating Professional Friction

In contrast to biopsychiatry, where the residents mastered patients' symptoms, diagnoses, and medication dosages and effects, psychotherapeutic competence revolved around distinct epistemic repertoires. As they approached the end of their training in talk and behavioral treatments, the residents were better equipped to showcase just such competence. They could ably identify patients' unrealistic thoughts or misguided behaviors and their concrete solutions in CBT. And they could skillfully discuss patients' inner conflicts and their manifestations in the treatment relationship in psychodynamic psychotherapy. In addition to showcasing their new skills, such performances enabled the residents to shed the constraints of psychotherapeutic novicehood and inhabit the status of initiates, mitigating some of the professional friction in their roles.

COMPETENCE IN COGNITIVE BEHAVIORAL THERAPY

The residents had an accelerated path toward competence in CBT because of its affinities with biopsychiatry. Within months of beginning this training, they could ably identify the specific cognitive, behavioral, and affective manifestations of patients' illnesses, along with the appropriate CBT tools and techniques necessary for treatment. Despite a less immersive training experience, they could skillfully perform CBT doctoring roles in group conversations, during role-plays, and in sessions with patients.

Making Sense of Patients' Worries in a CBT Framework

Much of the residents' training in CBT focused on teaching them to identify and counter patients' unrealistic thoughts and assumptions. And while earlier in their training the residents had unanticipated difficulties doing so, with time, they became increasingly adept at unraveling the constellations of thoughts, feelings, and behaviors that motivated patients' symptoms. During one midrotation meeting of the CBT for anxiety group, Jeremy, the instructor, along with the residents and the social work trainees, spent the better part of their time together discussing the case of Chris, a patient in treatment with Jennifer, one of the master of social work (MSW) fellows. Chris was an ardent Catholic with a strong sense of right and wrong who had begun to spend long periods praying. His behaviors were so debilitating that his family, also religious, had insisted he seek treatment. Jeremy invited the group to hypothesize about how the patient might explain his behaviors to himself. What motivated his extensive praying? If the group could elaborate some workable hypotheses, they would get closer to crafting a "cognitive restructuring" intervention.

Ely, still in his third postgraduate year at the time, excelled during the conversation. When someone proposed that perhaps Chris believed he had been chosen by God to be held to a higher standard than those around him, Ely asked, "What makes him different in the eyes of God? [. . .] He seems to be saying that the rules are different for him than for other people. Why is that?" This, Jeremy proposed, was a "viable thread" of inquiry. The resident had opened up a promising path for identifying and challenging Chris's beliefs. Building on Ely's hypothesis, Jeremy spelled out just how unrealistic such an expectation would be: "God would have to [. . .] pick [Chris] out, select him from all the millions of others." Next, God would have to "make a determination that [Chris] would have to be held to a higher salvation bar, determine that salvation bar, and then what? Monitor him." The case seemed airtight. "Does that seem like that would be on the top of God's list?," Jeremy asked, rhetorically.

But Jeremy had enough experience to know that the patient would not be so easily convinced. Leaving the inquiry on that triumphant note would miss the potential objections the patient could (and likely would) raise. The trainees would have to push their psychotherapeutic imaginations further, identifying Chris's possible doubts. Ely again demonstrated his skill, working out Chris's potential responses by drawing on his own religious knowledge: "Sometimes people feel like they are called by God and he might feel like that. . . . Certainly, the scripture has examples of that." And, Ely continued, Chris "could view his guilt and anxiety as the Holy Spirit working on him." Jeremy agreed: "Yeah . . . so he might say, 'in fact, my pain is a clear indication from God that this is in place!'" He encouraged further hypothesizing:

> *Jeremy (Instructor)*: What else might he say? What else might come after the "but"?
> *Jennifer (MSW)*: He's disappointed and he focuses his guilt on himself . . .
> *Jeremy*: Yeah, that's a good one. . . . "I get it, it's me, it's my internal thing that I have to be just right."
> *Ely (PGY-3)*: His standard's higher than God's!
> *Jeremy*: Yeah, higher than God's! Perfect! Thinking like a real CBT guy there! That's beautiful!

The building blocks of a convincing rebuttal—how could Chris's standards exceed God's own?—were set. Ely expanded on Jennifer's suggestion to establish the precise way in which the patient's expectations were "unreasonable." During the exercise, he established his CBT competence both by helping identify Chris's symptom-related thoughts and by pinpointing his possible objections to a therapist's rebuttal. In a treatment focused on reasoned discourse aimed at undoing patients' unreasonable thoughts, Ely showed his conversational dexterity. That Chris was not there to opine on the resident's suggestions was of little consequence: Ely had been able to display his CBT skill, "thinking like a real CBT guy." He had shown himself to be more than an ignorant novice, inhabiting instead the role of competent partner in the quest to figure out Chris's troubles and treatment.

Displaying CBT Skill and Self-Reflexivity during Role-Play

Role-plays were particularly effective platforms for the residents to establish their CBT competence. During these exercises, the residents could showcase their skills at identifying thoughts they could target with CBT techniques and implementing treatment approaches in a more uncertain interactional context relative to case discussions. Moreover, as opportunities for self-reflection and self-analysis, role-plays also enabled the residents to display their self-reflexivity. In the process, the residents established themselves as competent initiates, shedding their novice roles and demonstrating their ability to do CBT with little guidance from instructors.

Three months into the CBT for depression rotation, Robert, the instructor, invited the residents to try out CBT tools during role-play. In the exercise, Robert clarified, "the therapist would explain the CBT model" and the patient would "make it easy for [the partner] to apply the model." Turner (PGY-3) and Aaron (PGY-3) volunteered, the former playing the therapist and the latter the patient. Aaron had a ready problem to present—his anger at the conflicts stemming from having extended family living with him and his own family. Turner's task was to help Aaron work through these feelings. The role-play began with Aaron giving a brief explanation of his troubles:

Turner/Therapist: What are the things that have been going on?

Aaron/Patient: Things that I've been noticing in myself, is that I've been a lot more irritable lately, getting very angry and upset over small things that maybe previously didn't bother me?

Turner/Therapist: Most of those things are related to them [the extended family] being at home?

Aaron/Patient: Yeah, it's definitely related to that!

Turner/Therapist: If you think about those episodes of being angry and irritable, is there a particular thought that goes through your mind?

Aaron/Patient: Yeah, before I go home, I always have this thought, there's the expectation that the kitchen will be probably an absolute mess and I'll have to clean it . . .

Turner/Therapist: Sounds like you shouldn't be stuck in that situation of having to come home to a messy house. . . . I'd like to propose trying something today; there is something called cognitive behavioral therapy that is a technique that people can use without using any medication to try to improve your mood, and it's basically about trying to change the thoughts that you have, and talk back to yourself in a way that is more realistic. . . . So what we can do, is we can use this thought record, so I was gonna suggest to use this to talk about that event where you come home and you find a messy kitchen. . . . So when that happened, do you kind of remember what your feeling was at that moment?

Aaron/Patient: Yeah, like the feeling is the emotion? Yeah, it's like anger, frustration, which progressed into feeling depressed and sad . . .

Turner/Therapist: And the most intense one of them, which one do you think?

Aaron/Patient: Probably the anger . . .

Turner/Therapist: And you mentioned that the thoughts you had were "things shouldn't be that way." . . . Were there any other thoughts that you had?

Aaron/Patient: Yeah . . . like I shouldn't have to care for them, I'm not their parent, it's disrespectful . . .

Turner/Therapist: Which one of those is the most poignant for you?

Aaron/Patient: Probably the one saying I'm not their parents . . .

Turner and Aaron continued to work through the thought record, identifying alternative thoughts and feelings that Aaron could experience as he returned home. Turner had proven himself a capable therapist: he offered Aaron openings to elaborate on what he was experiencing, validated his feelings ("sounds like . . ."), explained the CBT model ("a technique that people can use . . ."), and oriented his partner toward working on particular thoughts. He had been able to, as Jason (PGY-4) put it, do "a good job of making it be a specific incident or a specific thought." Specificity is paramount in CBT, allowing therapists to work in targeted ways on their patients' unrealistic thoughts or symptom-driving behaviors. He had been "empathetic," Robert remarked, a key skill for getting a patient to collaborate in the work of treatment and give the therapist access to their inner life. In response, Turner admitted to facing some difficulties in therapy sessions "trying to understand what a patient is saying and also trying to fit it into a thought record." However, he told his colleagues, "having done it with patients a few times, it's been received well." His disclosure, coupled with his performance in the role-play, only served to solidify his competence.

But while Turner had done well enough, it was Aaron who excelled that day. His choice to draw on his own experiences opened up multiple possibilities for displaying his CBT know-how. For one, it allowed him to be an ideal patient, providing accurate and concrete accounts of his thoughts and feelings. Robert praised him: "I didn't expect you to choose your own thing, but I'm glad you did because that worked much better and you were able to give a lot more detail." Detail made for a successful role-play: Aaron had helped Turner achieve the specificity already noted by others in the group.

But drawing on his own experience also gave the resident an opportunity to display his skills as a therapist. During the discussion that followed,

Aaron told his colleagues that "when we talked about the anger and the thought in my head is that that turns against myself, and had we gone that way, we maybe would have done the vertical arrow technique" (a tool used to uncover patients' core beliefs about themselves). Taking the role of patient, he could speak from that "perspective" and see when meanings get lost in interaction. From his position, he knew that what he told and ultimately worked on with Turner was only a partial reflection of what he actually thought. The exchange, Aaron contended, could have taken a different turn had he been able "to get a point across" about his "anger," and had Turner "received" it more accurately. By invoking the "vertical arrow technique" as an alternative to the exercises he had just completed, Aaron showcased his CBT repertoire and his competence in the approach.

Finally, Aaron also shared with his colleagues: "You kind of use it [CBT] on yourself a lot of the times, and I do this with the DBT [dialectical behavioral therapy] mentorship as well, where I get into this situation and you recognize the thoughts, and I find myself supplying the alternative thoughts." In disclosing his self-work, Aaron was doing precisely what Robert had encouraged the residents to do: apply the tools to themselves as a way of learning and internalizing them. The resident went on to offer a version of the professional testimonials that helped in the collective management of skepticism, sharing that, having applied the techniques to himself, he "can see [. . .] how that can stem the effects of depression."

Aaron's message was clear: when properly used by an open-minded patient/resident, CBT techniques work. His self-reflexivity and conviction buttressed his overall performance: he had been a good patient and a good therapist, compellingly displaying CBT competence. It is important to note that neither he nor Turner had appealed to Robert for help during the exercise. They showed themselves to be capable CBT initiates who could take what they had learned and implement it in a self-directed way. No longer novices, the residents established their credibility as professionals with an expanded epistemic repertoire.

Successfully Navigating a Challenging Treatment and a Patient's Doubts in Session

Channeling patients during role-play and talking about their problems in clinical case discussions were sufficient bases for the residents to establish their competence. After all, the residents were infrequently (if ever) directly observed conducting psychotherapy. However, when such opportunities arose, their competence became more nuanced, including skills at carefully listening to and interacting with patients, strengthening the therapeutic relationship, and orienting patients toward doing CBT despite their resistance. Though these may not seem like CBT-specific skills, they were nevertheless deemed essential in this modality.

I introduced Sonora, a resident completing her fellowship in child psychiatry, in chapter 3, where I described her early struggles treating Sam, a young man who had come to the clinic at the urging of his family to address behavior that they thought was indicative of obsessive-compulsive disorder (OCD). The treatment lasted for nearly five months, and it remained a source of frustration and puzzlement for the resident, the other trainees, and Miriam, the experienced clinician who served as their instructor.

One of the main sources of exasperation for Sonora and her colleagues was Sam's inability or, as she would come to think, his unwillingness, to complete the homework exercises they crafted together every week and that were deemed essential to his betterment in this orientation. Two months into the treatment, Sonora shared with her colleagues that she "was getting annoyed" with Sam. "It's funny, I went home," she continued, "and I felt really irritable, really edgy . . . and I was like, I need to go run on my treadmill! And on Thursdays he's the only patient I see. . . . I think part of it was my interaction with him!" Sonora's admission earned her the group's empathy. It was also an implicit display of competence: as the treatment was becoming increasingly challenging, she had the self-awareness and the skills to temper the effects of her ill feelings.

Sonora's self-reflexivity became evident again as the group debated how she should talk to Sam about his reasons for not completing the CBT exercises. As her colleagues suggested lines of inquiry, Sonora cautioned, "I have to be conscious of the fact that I'm not too 'What are you doing, you slug!?'" She knew that she had to walk a tightrope, pushing Sam to engage more in the therapy while maintaining the rapport they had built. She could not sound too harsh in session. Her "annoyance" and "irritation" could not show. As soon as their session was under way, Sonora addressed Sam's lack of engagement head-on. Shortly after they started, she asked her patient whether he had "come up with any fabricated stories," as they had agreed he should during their previous session. Sam admitted he had not, and Sonora used this to discuss his expectations of treatment. After some back-and-forth, Sam revealed his doubts about the approach. Sonora pushed on:

> Sonora (PGY-4): When you say it's not too important, what do you mean, like, why bother doing it?
> Sam (Patient): Or like, why get my anxiety high to make it go lower?
> Sonora: So you feel like the whole concept of it is funny, 'cause it's, like, foreign to you?

Sam: Yeah . . . and it's kind of like . . .

Sonora: Uncomfortable . . .

Sam: Uncomfortable, and it's like a contradiction . . .

Sonora: You know what, it is a contradiction, and this therapy is different from other therapies!

Sonora had guided Sam toward a discussion of his difficulties in treatment. Her clarifying questions helped the patient share his doubts about their approach. She helped him articulate his thoughts and validated his doubts. And, having identified his skepticism, she could address it directly. The resident then spent the better part of the session doing so, moving closer to understanding Sam's expectations and his troubles:

Sonora (PGY-4): So you said that you thought this would go faster. Do you have a sense of why this isn't going faster?

Sam (Patient): I thought it would be easier . . .

Sonora: That's really the crux of it. This isn't easy . . . and I recognize that, and I know this isn't easy, it's not easy to talk about stuff, but we promised we'd be doing ERP [exposure and response prevention], not that it would be easy. . . . Because the anxiety, the depression is not easy either . . . or is it?

Sam: The depression is easy . . .

Sonora: What do you mean?

Sam: It's easier to stay in the depression . . .

Sonora: Yeah, so sometimes that happens, that it's comfortable here . . . stuck. . . . But there are other things you want, and it's hard to get to those goals . . . do you agree?

Sam: Yeah . . .

Sonora: So part of this is how do we get out of this? So it's gonna take work . . . it's not easy. [. . .] But the end result is that it does start helping with this stuff . . . and once you start, it does get easier to do things. . . . We're kind of stuck at this beginning step, right?

The resident held her frustration in check. She gently confronted Sam and opened a space for him to discuss his illness experience. Even when she reminded Sam of their task ("we promised we'd be doing ERP, not that it would be easy"), she did so while enabling him to share his own experiences. When she asserted that "the anxiety, the depression, is not easy," she checked herself, immediately asking her patient, "or is it?" Instead of assuming knowledge of his inner life, Sonora channeled psychotherapeutic uncertainty. She also reframed Sam's being "stuck" in the depression as "we're stuck" in the treatment, strengthening their alliance. By the end of the session, Sonora and Sam were coming up with his homework, "fabricated stories," together, the patient enthusiastically proposing scenarios that revealed his aspirations. The next time they met, Sam returned having partially completed his homework, a victory in a treatment that upended Sonora's expectations about CBT doctoring.

Sonora had shown herself to be a skilled therapist. Her competence was not only apparent to me. That she had done well became evident in the brief group conversation following the session. Sonora's colleagues praised her for getting "a lot done in an hour" and having "a good session." They remarked on her approaching Sam as "an ally," not "confrontational" as she had worried during their earlier conversation. One of the MSW fellows noted, "The way [Sonora] asked the questions, she never said 'You're not doing the homework,' but [the patient] still had to talk about why he wasn't [doing it]." Sonora's therapeutic skills came through in how she talked with Sam about his expectations of treatment, how she formulated her questions, how she shifted her tone from empathetic to playfully challenging. She could not force her patient to change. Instead, she offered a vivid demonstration of what famed CBT clinician Judith Beck called "the art of therapy," working with her patient collaboratively while also nudging him to work on himself.[1] To her audience behind the one-way mirror, the resident's difficulties and her success overcoming them made for compelling evidence of her competence. It was also a reminder that Sonora was no longer a novice, unsure of how to direct a treatment with a reluctant patient. Indeed, during the session she was a competent initiate, confidently guiding her patient toward implementing a CBT intervention.

COMPETENCE IN PSYCHODYNAMIC PSYCHOTHERAPY

While the residents' relational skills were important in CBT, they took on new meaning in psychodynamic psychotherapy. Here, their competence revolved around making sense of patients' feelings and connecting them to narratives about their internal and relational problems. All the while, the residents had to be attuned to their own roles in constituting treatment dynamics. These skills could not be any more different from what the residents learned in biopsychiatry, and it took almost the entirety of their time in psychodynamic training to develop them. In the psychodynamic rotation, the residents displayed their abilities in case presentations, where, with the aid of process notes, they could demonstrate their careful attention to the relational dynamics of treatment and their skills at navigating emotionally loaded moments in sessions. During group discussions, the residents also showcased their self-reflexivity. I describe how each of these dimensions of competence emerged during one particularly convincing case presentation by a resident nearing the end of his training.

Displaying Competence by Highlighting a Treatment's Relational Dynamics

Halfway through the first year of my observations, Jake, a PGY-4 weeks away from graduation, presented the case of Emily, a patient he had worked with for the better part of his two years in psychodynamic training. Jake began with a brief introduction:

> So just a quick reminder, she's a woman who lives [nearby] with her husband and her two kids. She's a homemaker there, she's got a medical history of some psychosomatic syndromes, but not much else. She first met our clinic through the evaluation clinic in August [. . .] when her PCP [primary care physician] referred her for anxiety. She's been in weekly psychotherapy with a focus being on conflict relating to her unfulfilled marriage, conflict about her sense of motherhood, more and more dilemmas about sexuality and sexual development and its relationship to her marriage and her womanhood, and then some erotic transference onto the therapist.

Jake's initial presentation skillfully framed the treatment, setting the tone for his presentation. He offered an abbreviated medical history but primed his audience by focusing on psychodynamically pertinent topics: the patient's inner "conflicts" about her identity and her domestic life, and how these conflicts came up in the treatment relationship through "some erotic transference onto the therapist," to borrow Jake's technical phrasing.

Before proceeding to read from his process notes, the resident described a recent breakthrough in the treatment that stemmed from a weather-related session cancellation. The patient, Jake told his colleagues, was "furious at the clinic for having canceled [the] appointment." She had disclosed her feelings during a phone conversation she had initiated, despite being "very reluctant to telephone [him] for fear of being an annoying, irritating, intrusive patient." Emily was, in Jake's telling, "growing in her capacity to tolerate more affect" and expressing it to him, a sign of improvement. During their next session, the resident explained, she engaged in "a healthy demonstration of anger" and "through the process, she was able to also acknowledge the fact that she was angry at [Jake]."

The resident's description of Emily's emotional expressions was not simply constitutive of a psychodynamic narrative about her troubles—it also functioned as testimony to the quality of their work. The patient's progress was reflected by her improved ability to "tolerate" a wider range of feelings and share them with her therapist—a sign that, instead of repressing difficult feelings, she could express them. Implicitly, Jake was also signaling that the therapeutic relationship was strong and trusting enough for Emily to experience this affective openness.

But it was not Emily's openness toward feelings in general that was most significant here. It was also the fact that she had begun to voice her feelings toward Jake that made the resident's presentation a compelling display of psychodynamic competence. By beginning with a description of Emily's feelings toward him, Jake brought the therapeutic relationship into focus. He continued:

> Then in late February and March, two separate occasions, she missed her appointments. That was because [of] two separate absences on my part that were discussed ahead of time, but they came within a three-week period. There was a one-week absence, we met, and the following week again I was away. So when I came back from that absence it was very clear there was a bit of a shift of focus on what she would bring up and those missed appointments, those absences, including the one that was due to the weather, made her really start to reflect in an experiential way on what it was gonna be like when therapy ended. And that's the language she has consistently used, so it's not 'what am I gonna do when you leave,' it's *it's ending*, our relationship is ending [Jake's emphasis].

The resident brought up a typical scenario: the therapist has to cancel appointments and the patient reciprocates in kind. As he discussed these sessions and stressed Emily's evocative language (e.g., "it's not 'what am I gonna do . . .'"), Jake showcased his psychodynamic understanding of her desires and her difficulties. For the resident, doctoring psychodynamically meant framing his own and Emily's missed sessions as meaningful "absences" that served as signposts as they worked through the end of their relationship. In invoking such relational dynamics and connecting them with the patient's progress along the path to self-insight, Jake had already demonstrated his skill in constructing a psychodynamically meaningful narrative about his treatment with Emily. He had also begun to show himself to be a competent observer of his patient's emotional states, an ability that became increasingly evident as Jake began to read from his process notes.

Competently Navigating Emotionally Charged Session Dynamics

Having started the presentation with a mention of the classic psychoanalytic theme of "erotic transference onto the therapist," Jake read a part of a session that would best fill in the empirical details for his audience. His choice of session, as will soon become apparent, further attested to his psychodynamic skill, being especially well suited to illuminating the dynamics of the treatment relationship. He started by mentioning Emily's punctuality ("she came in right on time, as usual"), a behavior that psychotherapists take as a positive sign of patients' investment in their treatments. Then, for several minutes, he read from the typed pages he had brought along, granting the group a retrospective view into an emotionally charged session. Shortly after he began reading, the resident remarked, "I don't quite do justice to her voice; she speaks very softly, and slowly, and timidly. So I'm gonna sound more casual than she does." In offering this comment, Jake was implicitly showcasing his careful observations of his patient's demeanor, giving additional dimension to his psychodynamic competence.

The appointment started with the patient discussing the visit of an out-of-town friend in whom she had confided the attraction she felt toward her therapist. The session then veered into a lengthy conversation about the impending end of treatment, and I include an extended excerpt of Jake's reading from his process notes:

Jake/Patient: I mean I know what's gonna happen in June, you will leave me, it'll stop there, it'll happen. But emotionally I don't know what I'm gonna do. [*Jake (PGY-4), interjecting his own description of the action into the narrative: She takes a pause here.*] What am I going to do if I need you? You're going to be off at your new job, with new people, new patients, other patients, I'll still want you, you'll forget about me. I'll know you don't want me, that you never wanted me, I know that now.

[*Jake (PGY-4): She starts to cry. I stay silent, she collects herself. She says:*]

Jake/Patient: This is so silly, it's ridiculous! It's embarrassing! I'm pathetic! But I'm going to miss you!

[*Jake (PGY-4): She's again trying to fight back tears.*]

Jake/Therapist: It looks as if you're in pain, the tears keep bubbling up, but you won't let them come.

[. . .]

Jake/Patient: I don't like it! I mean, I don't feel in control! It's weird, but it doesn't feel like it used to.

Jake/Therapist: I'm not sure I know what you mean by that.

Jake/Patient: During the past few sessions, I don't worry as much about crying. I mean, I still worry, just not as much.

Jake/Therapist: And what do you feel today in here when you cry?

Jake/Patient: Actually I like it. Sorry, that sounds weird. I mean, I almost feel comfortable. It's surprising. I feel more comfortable in here with you when I cry. I used to be so afraid that if I cried, you wouldn't comfort me, but I know that logically that's not supposed to happen. It's just that emotionally I feel stuck. There's this part of me that's been awakened in therapy and [. . .] I'm going to lose her . . .

Jake/Therapist: You're sad about my leaving you, but also that you might lose part of yourself? You're sad about two things.

Jake/Patient: Yeah . . . I mean, who's going to awaken that side of me if you're gone? I'm going to lose her.

Jake/Therapist: You mean this side of you? This side of you only has the capacity to come out when I'm around? It only comes out in therapy?

Jake/Patient: That's what I'm afraid of.

Jake/Therapist: So you're both sad and afraid.

[. . .]

Jake/Therapist: It sounds like the pain is about [. . .] intimacy, about a relationship. In your relationship with me you say you feel comfortable now with your tears. You keep fighting them off, though. Are you already feeling the pain that you're afraid of feeling in June?

Jake/Patient: Yes. Yes! [*Jake (PGY-4): She starts crying again.*] And I don't want to.

Jake/Therapist: You don't want to, yet at the same time you're afraid of losing our relationship.

Jake/Patient: Yes.

Jake/Therapist: Have you considered the possibility that maybe it's OK to feel sad before our last session? That you may feel more comfortable, to use your word, to cry and feel the pain while we're still together, while we still have the time to talk about it.

Jake/Patient: I don't know. Maybe.

As Jake read from his process notes, the emotional intensity of the session seemed palpable in the room. At times, members of the group gasped or laughed at some seemingly shocking answer or comment. I typed as quickly as I could, intuitively grasping that I was witnessing something important. Jake had chosen an evocative session and helped his audience understand it by filling in details about his and his patient's embodied demeanor. His process notes were replete with evidence of his psychodynamic skills. He showed himself to be an attuned observer of Emily's states and an able interlocutor for her spoken and unspoken expressions. He also showcased his skills at navigating the emotional currents flowing through the session. As I reread my notes, I was struck by his productive comments and self-control as Emily worked to articulate her feelings about the therapy and the therapist. While Emily expressed desires that exceeded the bounds of the typical doctor-patient relationship, Jake seemed calm, exhibiting the unruffled demeanor that experienced psychoanalysts deemed essential for fostering patients' own affect.

As he described it, Jake had found himself in the thick of *erotic transference*, a treatment dilemma that figures prominently in psychodynamic and psychoanalytic clinical practice: a patient turns their therapist into an object of desire by constructing a partial but idealized version of them as someone who can meet the patient's emotional needs.[2] While the situation can be (wrongly) flattering to the inexperienced clinician, it is described as "one of the most challenging phenomena" for therapists to navigate.[3] Jake was not alone in facing this conundrum, as other residents, both men and women, had described their own encounters with such dilemmas. Their experiences with patients' (more or less platonic) love confirmed that they were traversing an entirely different clinical terrain, one in which the doctor-patient relationship is not simply a conduit of empathy and treatment but also of deeper, more intimate, feelings. In such circumstances, the residents' competence depended on how well they navigated these charged relations in sessions and how they made sense of them psychodynamically. During the ensuing group discussion, Jake's performance of psychodynamic competence would be complete as he revealed his thinking about the treatment.

Showcasing Competence in the Discussion and Analysis of the Case

The process notes had revealed Jake to be a disciplined presence in the therapy room. The conversation that followed illuminated his psychodynamic thinking about his patient and, just as important, about himself. After the resident finished reading his process notes, a lively discussion ensued. The residents were eager to make sense of Emily's troubles and of Jake's own strategies for navigating such affectively charged work. The more experienced residents, Jake's cohort mates, offered counteranalyses to Jake's own. But these only became opportunities for Jake to bolster his psychodynamic competence. A key point of disagreement centered on Emily's understanding of "intimacy."

> *Jake (PGY-4)*: Intimacy is being a dutiful wife. [*Patricia (Instructor) murmurs in agreement.*] And that means taking care of the kids and [. . .] acquiescing to sex when her husband wanted sex. She never . . . she was always passive and never knew that it could be anything other than that . . .
>
> *Gordon (PGY-4)*: Other than this . . . But there's no, like, emotional aspect to her understanding of intimacy . . .
>
> *Jake*: Well, her belief is that she should be experiencing the emotional aspect of intimacy through all that. And therein is her conflict.
>
> *Patricia (Instructor)*: Um-hm.
>
> *Terry (Instructor)*: But she doesn't know what intimacy is.

Jake: She's not fulfilled in the marriage and says, this marriage has all the things that I believe a good intimate marriage should have, but why do I feel unfulfilled, and why am I experiencing this sexual awakening with my therapist . . .

Gordon: So then, when she starts developing emotional intimacy with you, does she characteristically sexualize the content to . . . address her discomfort with the affect involved in being emotionally intimate with you?

Jake: So it's a great point. So oftentimes . . . if she starts to get upset, and this has been happening recently. So we're talking explicitly now about termination and her grief. . . . She's doing a pretty good job processing it; however, every once in a while in a session, she'll kind of have what looks like an internal dialogue, lose her train of thought, and when I ask her where her train of thought went because her tears are now drying up, she's starting to have a fantasy about me. And so what she's learning is that her mind is defending against genuine, intense, sad emotion, by sexual fantasy. [*Patricia (Instructor)*: Um-hm.] And so she's recognizing that pattern in herself now, so there's that manifestation of I think what you're alluding to . . .

The exchange solidified Jake's performance of psychodynamic skill. Without hesitation, he described the workings of Emily's mind, identifying her unconscious "conflict" by drawing a contrast between her dedication to being a "dutiful wife" and the lack of "emotional [. . .] intimacy" she experienced. He justified his interpretation of Emily's troubles by appealing to his clinical experience treating her, and built on Gordon's own alternative psychodynamic framing. All the while, Patricia quietly offered validation. She needn't have done more: her relative silence was testimony to Jake's own abilities. The resident was no longer a novice in need of his instructors' input. He confidently offered his own psychodynamic interpretations, inhabiting the role of competent initiate.

But Jake's competence also hinged on a demonstration of self-reflexivity, and the residents were eager to learn about their colleague's own feelings in such an emotionally charged treatment. This would have been relatively unusual in biopsychiatry, where the feelings that garnered attention were largely patients' own. Yet being able to identify and discuss one's own feelings—along with those of one's patients—is a mark of competence in psychodynamic training. Jake made clear that his work with Emily had prompted much self-examination:

Sawyer (PGY-4): So how would, I'm just curious, how would being in a . . . you know . . . The only difference in the therapeutic relationship is, you know, you're not gonna flirt with her, and have sex with her [. . .] but,

I mean, you're . . . She must know that you have ideas or thoughts of
her . . .

Jake (PGY-4): She [. . .] deeply wants to know my thoughts about her. And
she's hopefully coming to some knowledge that as a man I might have
very biologically rooted reactions to her, as an attractive woman, that
I might find her attractive [. . .]. But that I'm not going to, so that I can
have a fantasy world, but not act on it. Whereas she doesn't separate
fantasy from reality. Every time she'll tell me about a fantasy of mine,
she'll then profusely apologize . . .

Terry (Instructor): You talking about a fantasy of yours or . . . ?

Jake: A fantasy of me . . . sorry . . .

[*Laughter in the room as Jake seems embarrassed by the slip.*]

Jake [*animatedly*]: You see what I'm saying, though? She'll say, "That's so
intrusive," as if she had done that to me. So if she had a fantasy about
touching me and she told me about it, that was the same thing as having
touched me.

The lines between fantasy and reality, and those between patient and
therapist, were not always easy to maintain. In the context of psychodynamic psychotherapy, such boundaries took on new significance, and the
residents were persistently encouraged to turn the analytic lens toward
just such difficulties and the reactions they stirred up. Jake chose his
words carefully as he made clear that having a "fantasy world" was not
solely the domain of patients. Yet what therapists can do, and what Jake
did, is "not act on it"—both for ethical and for treatment reasons. Jake
was modeling relationship-appropriate intimacy to his patient, and his
efforts were beginning to pay off in the treatment. Emily was becoming
increasingly able to tell that she was blurring the boundaries between
personal and professional, between fantasy and reality, "recognizing that
pattern in herself now." In psychodynamic terms, Jake's self-discipline
was fostering Emily's insight.

Whatever the effects of Jake's self-reflexivity on the treatment, the
group discussion showcased his abilities both in and out of the treatment
room. As he neared his final meeting with Emily, his self-discipline was
becoming increasingly important. Zoli (PGY-3), a junior resident at the
time, echoed a concern that had come up earlier in the conversation:

Zoli (PGY-3): I think one thought that I had, and it's more about the frame,
as you guys are ending and working with your supervisor about this,
like some of the times you presented material [. . .] how at one point it
was so eroticized. [. . .] And I think something about a hug, [. . .] but
obviously how one goodbyes . . . a handshake, "so long!"

Patricia (Instructor): You must anticipate it, absolutely!

Zoli: [. . .] That brings a little bit of anxiety . . . just how to . . .

Jake: Absolutely! In fact, I've experienced some anxiety about that in recent weeks, and talking to my supervisor about it . . . 'cause I was eager to get some advice on [that. . . .] This is gonna be a woman who . . . may want some sort of physical contact as a piece of closure, but also she's struggling a little bit now with desperation, and there's at least one moment in each session now. . . . The sessions in general are much more productive . . . are less about sex, they're really about just grieving over the loss of therapy and moving on [. . .]. But, there's at least a moment in every session where she's like, you know, "Maybe I should just go for it, what do I have to lose, therapy's ending, maybe I should just come over there and . . ."

Vinit (PGY-4): She's saying that out loud?

Jake: Yeah, yeah!

[*Vinit gives a small laugh.*]

Patricia: It's good that she'll say it out loud; it's actually harder to deal with when it's silent.

Jake's "anxiety" was not unfounded: Emily was contemplating a breach in the therapeutic frame. His colleagues validated his concerns and suggested solutions. Leah (PGY-3) wondered whether Jake "should [. . .] have a camera in the room to protect [himself]," and Vinit (PGY-4) advised a room with a "one-way mirror." Observability took on new meaning as the residents worried about the potential implications of a situation in which Emily would initiate physical contact. Yet Jake once again deployed his psychodynamic know-how to make sense of the situation, mirroring Patricia's final comment. Even as he worried about possible physical contact, he reiterated, "I'm glad that even when she has these impulses, she's still bringing them up." He had not always been that confident. "There was a time," Jake told his colleagues, "when I was, like, what am I gonna do if she comes on to me, you know?" However, he was "past that point in [his] own countertransference." Jake's clinical experience and self-knowledge amounted to a renewed sense of professional assurance.

As the group conversation drew to a close, it became clear that one of Jake's remaining tasks was to find a new therapist for Emily. The treatment, done for Jake, would continue—or start over—for his patient. But the resident's competence was not diminished by his seeming failure to "cure" Emily. His case presentation contained all the elements of psychodynamic skill: he paired evocative process notes with insightful analysis and matched the attention he paid to his patient with his own clear-eyed self-reflexivity. The resident had successfully enacted a psychodynamic therapeutic role. That he could also show his patient's own growing insight into her troubles and unconscious dynamics was welcome testimony to his effectiveness as a psychodynamic therapist.

Allaying Epistemic Friction and Developing New Doctoring Repertoires

As the residents became increasingly competent in CBT and psychodynamic psychotherapy, they also began to accommodate these approaches into their existing biopsychiatric repertoires. No longer keeping psychotherapeutic techniques and ideas at arm's length, they instead found ways to expand their doctoring approaches by incorporating them into their day-to-day work. Most frequently, the residents turned to *pragmatic accommodation*, making use of pharmacological or talk and behavioral tools as they saw fit. CBT was particularly amenable to such practices, and I briefly describe below how the residents accomplished this with their patients. A deeper integration occurred when they attempted to enact *hybrid repertoires*, assimilating their psychotherapeutic, typically psychodynamic, skills and ideas into their biopsychiatric tool kit.

PRAGMATIC ACCOMMODATION

The residents had no shortage of reasons to turn to psychotherapy in their work with patients. Zoli (PGY-3) shared with his colleagues in the interpersonal psychotherapy (IPT) rotation: "My experience in depression has been limited, [but] a lot of folks I see are chronic. And as a clinician you feel helpless about that, but at the same time you want to offer something, so it becomes all about 'Let's try this med, and then that med.'" The resident knew that being a competent doctor meant that he could not betray his "helplessness" to his patients. Instead, wanting to "offer something," he would resort to "trying" various "meds"—alas, to no avail. Psychotherapy was a workable alternative. Zoli explained that he had "seen a lot of success, especially with CBT" and that he was eager to learn new therapeutic techniques.[4] As he offered professional testimony about the benefits of CBT, he also revealed his expanding epistemic repertoire and pragmatic use of it.

About three months into the CBT for depression rotation, Turner (PGY-3) told the group about a patient who had come to psychiatric emergency services (PES) "very distressed." Yet, Turner explained, "I couldn't give him any benzoates, and I was, like, 'Fuck, what can I do?!'" Unable to rely on his core expertise and prescribe a psychiatric medication, the resident faced a treatment dilemma. The solution lay with his therapeutic training: "I taught him some deep breathing techniques and that was very helpful!" Turner and his patient had navigated their shared crisis with the aid of a CBT intervention. The resident had found a way forward through the pragmatic use of psychotherapeutic tools.

To be clear, whereas CBT was ideal for such moment-to-moment professional bricolage, psychodynamic psychotherapy also lent itself to pragmatic accommodation. Recall Ely, the resident whose journey from skeptical observer to competent practitioner of psychodynamic psychotherapy I traced in chapter 6. Toward the end of his residency training, he delivered a case presentation about his treatment with Nina, the patient who had eluded his efforts at establishing a productive psychodynamic treatment relationship by missing sessions and engaging in superficial talk when she did come to therapy. The resident began his presentation by melding a biopsychiatrist's attention to symptoms with a psychodynamic therapist's disregard for psychiatric diagnosis: Nina "came in through one of the clinics [and] I think her diagnosis was dysthymic disorder versus maybe double depression," he told the group. As for her symptoms, Ely (PGY-4) explained, "she had struggled with negative self-image, as well as neuro-vegetative stuff, [and] low energy."

To help with some of these symptoms, Ely "put her on some Celexa," and "she stabilized very quickly."[5] Though his psychoanalytic supervisor, Ely explained, "wasn't super big on me continuing the medications, there were no side effects, and so [Nina and I] quickly stopped talking about the medications [during sessions]," turning their attention instead to whatever Nina was willing to share. Ely had sidestepped his supervisor's advice and continued Nina's drug treatment, pragmatically mixing pharmacological and psychodynamic approaches. And though he was, as a result, occupying dual roles with respect to his patient, Ely deemed the arrangement "at least in the session [. . .] not a big issue." For patient and resident, the matter of mixing biopsychiatric and psychodynamic approaches seemed settled: the former would serve a supporting role for the latter, in an arrangement reminiscent of medications' initial introduction into the psychoanalytically dominated psychiatry of the 1960s.

HYBRID REPERTOIRES

For a minority of the residents, a hybrid doctoring approach proved more epistemically and professionally productive. During a conversation we had toward the end of his training, Lucas (PGY-4) told me, "When patients come in telling me of increased symptoms, and I get this sense that they're looking for a medication solution," he asks himself, "Is this going to be an evidence-based use of medication or a reactive use of medication?" If a discussion with the patient reveals that "they're having some interpersonal or [. . .] a kind of meaningful conflict," Lucas explained, he tries to steer them away from medications. "There's no specific study that shows that, you know, 'I'm worried about [. . .] getting married again because my first marriage ended in shambles.' We don't really study whether citalopram helps for that."[6] For Lucas, this would mean that "just because [the prospect of marriage] happens to be causing anxiety or just because it happens to be causing sad feelings," that does not "mean necessarily that [a drug is] going to be helpful." Psychodynamic training allowed Lucas to discern whether patients' problems would be best served by medications or whether a nonchemical treatment would be warranted instead.

Parsing out the biological and psychological dimensions of patients' illness experiences was a primary preoccupation for residents who adopted such hybrid repertoires. Clara, a recent Shorewood graduate, spoke to me about this at length in her recently established private office. She was still setting things up, she told me, struggling with the dilemmas of starting a practice where she could prescribe medications *and* do psychotherapy. She was also contemplating psychoanalytic training. She told me, "As I got further along in my [residency] training, it seemed like though medications can be useful and there is definitely a biological basis to a lot of a person's symptomatology, it seems like what's going on in their life and what has gone on in their life also contributes a lot to the difficulties that they're having." Though "prescribing medications [. . .] is oftentimes what is expected now of a psychiatrist because," she said with a laugh, "we can!" Clara thought that "most times that's not enough." Instead, she thinks about patients' problems "more holistically." This hybrid approach seemed less a matter of practical choice and more of an intellectual commitment that Clara and other like-minded residents had made once they became competent in psychotherapy.

For Vinit (PGY-4), psychiatric and psychodynamic approaches were inseparable as he tried to make sense of a challenging treatment. During one of the psychodynamic group meetings, Vinit presented parts of an ongoing treatment with Dana, a patient who had come to the clinic seeking help with depression. Akin to Jake, Vinit had recently faced the challenge of managing the patient's cancellations following his own announced absence. When the resident and his patient were finally able to reconnect, Dana was aggrieved. "After some superficial discussion" during their first session back in treatment, the patient "started complaining about the fact that [Vinit] had said to increase her depression medication dose when what she really wanted was to decrease that dose and eventually get off the meds." Moreover, the patient thought, Vinit had also failed as a therapist. She wondered aloud, Vinit told his colleagues, "what the therapy is doing for her when [he is] just sitting there quietly, not saying anything."

Reading from his process notes, Vinit recalled Dana telling him, "I could just go home and talk to a wall and it would be cheaper!" This incited the residents' laughter. Some concurred with the patient's assessment of the financial benefits of "talk[ing] to a wall."[7] Vinit defended himself: "True, but I think I do a better job than a wall!"

The resident had created a compelling setup for what was to come. He had found himself in a nearly impossible situation with his patient early in the treatment, seemingly ineffective both biopsychiatrically and therapeutically. He would soon turn the conversation around. Vinit continued reading from his process notes:

> I'm listening to this and I'm not mad, but I want to try to defend myself a bit, and I said, "Based on my recollection, I remember you were unhappy with your PCP who suggested to stop the meds cold turkey." She said tearfully that she wanted to work on getting off the medication. [*Vinit returns to reading from his process notes of the conversation.*] "In all honesty, I was never aware of that preference that you had. I want to know why you asked for my opinion about what to do when you already had a preference with the meds?" Patient said that she needed reassurance that she was making the right decision.

The patient's desire for reassurance was, Vinit explained to the group, deeply rooted: "Her mom used to do that for her." Having begun his case presentation with the almost disastrous start of treatment—even his supervisor had thought the patient would stop coming to therapy—Vinit turned the narrative around, illuminating his abilities instead. For the next several minutes he discussed the treatment in psychodynamic terms, drawing out Dana's need for reassurance and his ability to foster her insight into how this manifested itself in her relationships. Not only had he managed to ease Dana back from the edge of quitting treatment, but he also found new ways to help her reflect on herself through the lens of the therapeutic relationship. For Vinit, this was a reframing of his doctoring role. Managing the patient's medications was not simply about symptoms and drug effects. It was also about the relationship that he and his patient were in the process of building. The resident could not do pharmacology without psychodynamic psychotherapy, and only by using them in tandem could he best help his patient. A hybrid repertoire enabled him to navigate the challenges of treatment.

Conclusion

Competence, sociologist Mary-Jo DelVecchio Good has argued, "is a core symbol in the culture of American medicine."[8] Medical practice and medical education center on assessing, contesting, and delivering competent doctoring performances. While early in medical school these center on formal and informal tests, later, case presentations, case discussions, and, in some instances, interactions with (sometimes surrogate) patients, become increasingly common.[9] Finally, as newly minted MDs enter the postgraduate years, they shift away from largely didactic assessments toward clinical contexts. Their competence depends on being able to understand patients' problems, formulate them in the terms of their specialization, and treat them with its tools, all the while managing the demands of hospital life and those of the senior physicians with whom they work.[10]

But although competence is "fundamental to the everyday clinical work and professional experience of American physicians," it is, DelVecchio Good notes, conceptually slippery.[11] Though we may know a competent doctor when we see one, it is hard to articulate precisely what makes her so. In the field of mental health, where cures are largely out of reach and treatments long-lasting, the problem of defining—and recognizing—competence is more acute. Indeed, the residents' instructors were attuned to these problems. In one instance, during the first day of the interpersonal psychotherapy rotation, Holly, the instructor, cautioned the residents, "We inadvertently develop a mode of thinking that we must help the patient be problem free, but there's nobody out there who does not have any problems whatsoever." For the residents, this meant that establishing competence is less about proclaiming patients cured—as useful as this might be in the collective management of skepticism—and more about their facility with the tools, skills, and assumptions of a given approach.

Competence is not simply a technical imperative. It is also a professional and moral one.[12] To echo DelVecchio Good, it encompasses both the "presentation of patients" and the "presentation of 'self.'"[13] Concerned with "transcending the role of student," medical trainees seek ways to display their professional judgment, all the while embodying respectable and legitimate selves.[14] For psychiatry residents, accustomed to doing so within a biopsychiatric framework, psychotherapeutic competence raised particular challenges that they managed, early on, by appeal to skepticism. Yet as they learned more about what it means to doctor in each of the talk and behavioral approaches, they had less use for doubt and could instead showcase new capable selves. For them, competence was thus also about fashioning resolutions to the contradictions that had defined their roles as therapy trainees.

While the professional and epistemic frictions in their roles did not entirely disappear, they did attenuate as the residents advanced in the program. With time and experience, the residents became better equipped to navigate such frictions. Professionally, they could rely on their advanced status and their knowledge of doctoring in diverse approaches to push back against the constraints of novicehood. They could confidently share their views on a particular patient's conundrums and implement a course of psychotherapeutic treatment with only minimal input from supervisors and instructors. Epistemically, the residents continued to confront the inherent contradictions between biopsychiatry and psychotherapy, but they fashioned their own resolutions through pragmatic accommodation or hybrid repertoires.

Pragmatic accommodation seemed to present the residents with fewer challenges. The approach allowed them to remain rooted in pharmacology and simply tap into their psychotherapeutic repertoire as needed. For these psychiatrists, psychotherapy became part of an expert "tool kit" of possible epistemic machineries, to be used as they adjusted their "strategies of action" in response to uncertain treatment conditions.[15] CBT lent itself best to such accommodation, its concrete techniques easier to incorporate into medication management sessions when pharmacological tools were of limited use. These doctors' professional identities remained rooted in biopsychiatry, with psychotherapy playing only an ancillary role in their work.

Less frequently, the residents adopted a hybrid approach that integrated biopsychiatric and psychotherapeutic epistemes. Those who did so found biological explanations of mental illness insufficient and were compelled to make sense of patients' troubles by alternative means. Unlike the pragmatic model, which left the residents' explanatory schemas intact, hybridity shifted their understandings of why patients suffered. These residents came to think that while some of their patients' symptoms could be explained biologically, their illnesses were better understood as the result of interactions between relational, psychological, and biological factors. For these psychiatrists, attending to the nonbiological dimensions of patients' suffering meant relying on the psychodynamic apparatus of assumptions and interventions.

These two forms of resolution—pragmatic and hybrid—made different demands on the residents' work and careers. Pragmatic accommodation did not require a radical shift in the residents' professional dispositions and practices, particularly when it entailed applying CBT in pharmacology appointments. Given that such accommodation consisted largely of employing specific CBT tools when drugs fell short, the practice made few additional temporal demands on the residents' work. Hybridity was more onerous, particularly when residents committed to doing psychodynamic psychotherapy with their patients. To put hybrid repertoires into practice, they had to set aside time for psychodynamic sessions and make an investment, material and temporal, into ongoing supervision. They also had to potentially forgo insurance reimbursement because insurers do not typically cover psychotherapy sessions at the same rate as pharmacological ones. Finally, they had to work with a smaller number of patients who could pay out of pocket. Hybridity was, decidedly, the more difficult epistemic and professional path.

8 * From Skepticism to Competence

AN INTEGRATED THEORY AND IMPLICATIONS

This book started out with a puzzle: how do psychiatry residents, firmly rooted in pharmacology, come to view psychotherapy as a legitimate and even, at times, preferable treatment for their patients' problems? Since the 1980s, the profession of psychiatry has become increasingly committed to a view of mental illness as a biological disease. This view has redefined its approach to research and treatment and reshaped the education of its practitioners. Yet starting in 2001, psychiatry residents have also been required to learn psychotherapy. Despite the significance of this shift for the field, we know little about how the requirement has been put into practice and what challenges, if any, those who must do so face. The previous pages have begun to fill this gap by offering an analysis of how psychiatry residents manage the dilemmas of learning to doctor without drugs.

During the final two years of the four-year residency, when much of their talk and behavioral training is clustered, the residents are caught between two competing worlds: biopsychiatry and psychotherapy. These worlds, however, do not exercise equal pull on their professional roles or epistemic imaginaries. Much of the residents' time and attention is dedicated to honing their pharmacological competence. Their professional identities come to be defined by the biological study and treatment of mental illness. But psychotherapy upends their expectations. In psychodynamic, cognitive behavioral therapy (CBT), and other talk and behavioral rotations, the residents learn that talking with patients can help not just in addition to but sometimes instead of prescribing medications. This book tells the story of the residents' conundrums as they navigate these new knowledge domains and new roles, and shows how they move from skepticism toward psychotherapy to competence in its various approaches.

The Preconditions, Management, and Resolution of Skepticism

Psychotherapy training places the residents in contradictory roles that are defined by epistemic and professional frictions. Such frictions in turn activate the inevitable skepticism associated with being compelled to learn something that contradicts one's existing beliefs and occupy less desirable positions. But contrary to what we might expect, the foregoing chapters have shown that skepticism is not simply a protective shell that closes off the possibility of developing new professional repertoires. Instead, in particular social conditions, skepticism becomes productive, enabling experimentation with different practices and roles and facilitating new forms of competence. Building on the residents' experiences, I offer an integrated theory that details skepticism's "social preconditions," to borrow Mary Douglas's formulation, as well as its collective management, and its resolution.[1]

THE "SOCIAL PRECONDITIONS" AND USES OF SKEPTICISM

Skepticism flourishes in social conditions marked by friction, role contradictions, and status threats. Unlike the medical students and other initiates who are the subjects of earlier writing on professionalization, the residents whose stories animate this book did not approach psychotherapy training as tabulae rasae. Instead, they came to it as already socialized professionals with their own assumptions about the organization of their field and their position in it. Whether it raised fundamental questions about where mental illness is located (i.e., the brain, the unconscious, or thoughts and behavior) or how it can be treated (i.e., chemically, through talk, or thinking and behavior modification), psychotherapy training challenged residents' expectations about what it means to doctor. In turn, the residents' existing knowledge about the biology of mental illness primed them to greet psychotherapeutic assumptions and practices with doubt.

But more than fostering such epistemic friction, psychotherapy training also resulted in professional friction and a perceived status threat for the residents. Their positions in the field of mental health are akin to those of "educated and privileged" elites who, as anthropologist Mary Douglas explained, turn to "radical" skepticism when "faced with unacceptable arbitrary power," and they are "helpless to challenge it."[2] Psychiatrists have long claimed privileged roles in the field of mental health, historically excluding psychologists and social workers from their core jurisdiction, such as in the superintendence of asylums, psychoanalysis, or, contemporarily, pharmacology.[3] The implicit promise the profession makes to its trainees is that, with sufficient education and time, they themselves can occupy such positions of power.[4] And while psychiatry residents begin to inhabit such roles during more advanced stages in their training, in psychotherapy they are compelled into novicehood vis-à-vis the psychologists and social workers who serve as their instructors. Even as psychotherapy training is partly premised on the assumption that, by learning talk and behavioral approaches, psychiatrists can continue to occupy leadership roles in multidisciplinary treatment teams, this is far from the residents' minds as they struggle with the contradictory demands of their roles. As professional novices subjected to supervision and oversight, skepticism becomes a convenient tool for residents wishing to shore up their doctoring worth and status.

Finally, the residents are powerless to change their training even if they view some aspects of it as "unacceptable" or "arbitrary," to use Douglas's phrasing. They must meet the requirements of the program and, implicitly, of the Accreditation Council for Graduate Medical Education (ACGME). The residents do push back against how these requirements are put into practice—by, for example, treating fewer patients in psychotherapy or meeting with them less frequently than their instructors and supervisors advise—but they are nevertheless beholden to carry them out to their superiors' satisfaction. The psychiatrists must develop at least a modicum of competence in psychotherapy if they wish to graduate and become board certified, even as they may not initially anticipate using psychotherapeutic techniques in their professional work.

Nevertheless, unlike the intellectual elites who, in Mary Douglas's analysis, embraced "radical skepticism" when they felt themselves subjugated and marginalized, the residents knew that their status as professional novices in psychotherapy was temporary. And, while early in their talk therapy training, skepticism served these psychiatrists as a protective shell that enabled them to maintain professional worth by appealing to biopsychiatric and clinical knowledge, later, this same skepticism allowed them to experiment with new ways to doctor without fearing a loss of status. This shift in skepticism's valence is not coincidental, nor can it be explained by a sudden transformation in the residents' minds. Instead, it is attributable to specific social conditions, and I turn to describing these next.

RELATIONAL CONTEXTS AND THE COLLECTIVE
MANAGEMENT OF SKEPTICISM

To better understand how the residents' skepticism became less defensive and more productive of new competencies, we must first account for the features of psychotherapy rotations that made this process possible. While the manifest function of psychotherapy meetings was to expose trainees to various therapeutic techniques and help them troubleshoot clinical conundrums, their latent purpose was to strengthen their belief in the value of psychotherapy. For this, the collective management of skepticism was essential. Left to their own devices, skeptics will simply echo one another's doubts, remaining in their ideational silos.[5] Psychotherapy group meetings had three dimensions that worked against such closure, fostering the residents' engagement with unfamiliar approaches: the meetings were organized around offering support and correction, they opened psychotherapeutic expertise up to witnessing, and they created avenues for low-stakes experimentation. I discuss each in turn.

First, group meetings functioned as the kind of "relational spaces" that organizational scholar Katherine Kellogg deemed essential for facilitating institutional change.[6] In group discussions, junior residents could express their uncertainties and, more important, their misgivings, to an audience of peers who struggled with similar challenges. In addition to recognition and validation, these same peers could offer assistance, helping their colleagues troubleshoot challenges and revealing paths toward therapeutic competence. The residents thus found in these conversations not only an echo chamber for their skepticism but also a way out of it. For their part, instructors did not dismiss the residents' doubts. They offered validation, along with corrections and advice when necessary. They also affirmed the residents' knowledge and status by asking for their input in case discussions and deferring to them on questions of pharmacology. Put simply, these meetings were spaces where the residents' existing knowledge was recognized, and their skepticism was affirmed and addressed.

Second, rotations also offered residents opportunities to witness psychotherapeutic expertise in action. As I have argued in chapter 4, drawing on the work of science and technology scholars, such witnessing serves a dual role: it makes apprenticeship possible by opening expertise up for observation, and it legitimates the practices rendered visible in the process. In psychotherapy rotations, the residents had opportunities to watch trusted instructors work with patients and hear them explain their approaches. They also got to see their more experienced colleagues' performance of therapeutic competence when they presented and discussed their own psychotherapeutic work, offering professional testimonials about its utility. Finally, they could see these same colleagues model distinct approaches to accommodating the contradictory demands of biopsychiatry and psychotherapy, revealing possible paths forward.

Third, group meetings were platforms for low-stakes experimentation with psychotherapeutic doctoring. Whether this meant contributing to case discussions, delivering case presentations, or participating in role-play, the residents got to inhabit psychotherapeutic roles and do so in supportive environments. This activity, in turn, compelled them to step out of the position of skeptical observers of psychotherapy and engage with CBT and psychodynamic approaches on their own terms. Crucially, the residents could do so without committing to becoming psychotherapists. Instead, they could temporarily inhabit therapeutic modes of talking, thinking, and interacting while remaining rooted in their biopsychiatric identities. They could try out psychotherapeutic repertoires knowing that these roles could be as temporary or as permanent as they wished.

In sum, skepticism's defensive function is attenuated in socio-relational conditions that facilitate the collective management of doubt. Settings where skeptics can express their doubts in the company of peers and have them validated and addressed ensure status maintenance even as closely held beliefs may be challenged. Additionally, skepticism can become productive when one witnesses trusted others engage with and put new ideas into practice. Finally, experimenting with new practices in low-stakes environments can foster new forms of competence without undermining skeptics' existing statuses. Together, validation, observation, and experimentation turn skepticism from an insulating shell into a safe and productive platform for developing new ideas and practices.

SKEPTICISM'S RESOLUTION AND THE DEVELOPMENT OF COMPETENCE

Skepticism's resolution need not amount to transformation, a complete reversal of beliefs, identities, or practices. Nor is the suspension of skepticism desirable.[7] Indeed, rendering skepticism productive rather than defensive may be preferable as it enables both critical and constructive engagement with differently positioned interlocutors. The relational contexts I outlined in the previous section are partly responsible for activating skepticism's productive dimension. Additionally, as Mary Douglas and Jason Owen-Smith both demonstrated, this shift is further enabled by participants' anticipated status gains.[8] But building from this more open, if still doubting, stance toward new competencies requires one additional step: that of self-reflexivity.

Early on, when the residents' knowledge of psychotherapy was minimal, and their positions vis-à-vis instructors and supervisors hewed closer to subordination, skepticism served to insulate their valued identities as biopsychiatrists. Through displays of doubt, they could project their doctoring worth in positions structured to undermine their existing status.[9] Yet skepticism did not close off engagement with psychotherapy altogether. Indeed, in the meetings of psychotherapy rotations, residents received validation and were offered opportunities for observation and experimentation. These conditions rendered their skepticism productive. This, in turn, enabled the residents' practical engagement with psychotherapeutic doctoring.

This pivotal stage in the residents' trajectories was marked by increased self-reflexivity. As they learned more about various talk and behavioral interventions and experimented with their application in group discussions or with patients, the residents also became increasingly attuned to the disjunctures between biopsychiatric and psychotherapeutic assumptions. In the company of peers and instructors, they began to acknowledge their limitations and engage with them productively, glimpsing new doctoring possibilities. Significantly, they started turning the analytical lens not only toward their doctoring roles but also toward their inner lives, reflecting and working on them with the tools they were learning. Expressions of doubt increasingly gave way to displays of self-reflexivity.

Implicitly, the residents shifted from skeptical observers of psychotherapy to engaged participants in their own psychotherapeutic socialization. This engagement, in turn, enabled new competencies. In CBT, the residents showcased their skills at disentangling thoughts from behaviors, feelings, and situations, and tailoring the orientation's interventions to patients' particular illness configurations. The residents also grew into more capable participants in role-plays, inhabiting each role within CBT parameters. In psychodynamic psychotherapy they skillfully reflected on patients' inner conflicts and the meanings of the therapeutic relationship. Finally, they competently drew out the largely unspoken emotional and relational dynamics of treatment and their own contributions to fostering them. In short, the residents became competent initiates in talk and behavioral therapies.

The consequences of psychotherapeutic competence for the residents' doctoring repertoires varied. Most turned toward pragmatic accommodation. For these doctors, pharmacology remained the primary mode of treatment, complemented by psychotherapy only when medications fell short. CBT, with its concrete tools and time-limited interventions, lends itself particularly well to such intermittent integration. In contrast, a small minority of residents incorporated their newfound psychotherapeutic competence into hybrid doctoring repertoires.[10] They transitioned toward deeper engagement with psychotherapy, particularly the psychodynamic approach, using it less as a set of tools to be deployed as needed and more as a durable disposition. Practically, such residents brought their nuanced epistemic repertoires to bear on patients' problems as they tried to discern whether pharmacology or psychotherapy would be the appropriate lens for understanding and treating them.

To be clear, there are powerful forces that work against psychiatrists' deeper commitment to psychotherapy, forces that, as I discuss later, residents who embraced the hybrid approach had to fight against. Their employers hire them to prescribe, insurers pay them when they do so, and patients frequently expect a prescription along with (or instead of) a listening ear. Put simply, psychiatrists are compelled to work as medication prescribers. But some also try to craft alternatives to this typical trajectory by pursuing additional training (typically psychoanalytic) or establishing private practices where they can conduct psychotherapy appointments.

In sum, though epistemic and professional frictions activate skepticism, relational contexts that facilitate validation, observation, and experimentation work against the entrenchment of doubt. As skepticism becomes productive, self-reflexivity and self-analysis supplant withdrawal and self-preservation, instead facilitating engagement with new ideas and practices. This, in turn, makes possible new competencies. Though none of the residents completely reversed their commitments to biopsychiatry, they did develop new fluency in psychotherapy. The frictions between these distinct approaches to mental illness did not disappear. Nor did the contradictions between being novices and professionals. But both attenuated, as the residents found new ways to integrate their seemingly antithetical doctoring mandates and anticipated their graduation from the program. Skepticism remained useful, not as a mode of defense but rather as one of engagement.

The Implications of Teaching Psychotherapy to Psychiatrists

To readers with even passing familiarity with contemporary psychiatry, the fact that residents have to learn psychotherapy at all may come as a surprise. This reaction would not be misplaced. A recent survey found that a little over half of American psychiatrists spend their time with patients prescribing medications without providing any psychotherapy.[11] Those who still include psychotherapy in their work do so in a minority of patient visits.[12] Psychiatry has become a profession whose practitioners are, by and large, dedicated to the chemical management of mental illness through psychiatric drugs. Yet this should not be taken for the disappearance of psychotherapy from psychiatry.[13]

The same survey found that the percentage of psychiatrists who continue to do psychotherapy exclusively has remained steady since the 1990s, hovering between 11 percent and 15 percent.[14] Moreover, practice guidelines from the American Psychiatric Association recommend a combination of drugs and psychotherapy across a range of diagnoses, and clinical research supports these recommendations.[15] Finally, as a result of changing accreditation standards in psychiatry and medicine more broadly, starting in 2001 psychiatry trainees have been required to develop competence not only in pharmacological treatments but also in psychodynamic and cognitive behavioral psychotherapies, the two approaches dominant today.[16] Despite earlier ruptures and persistent doubts, psychotherapy has remained a part of psychiatric training.

While this book focuses on how psychiatry residents navigate the conundrums of putting this organizational imperative into practice, the story it tells also offers new ways to think about psychiatric training, the psychiatric profession, and its role in the broader field of mental health. In the following pages, I propose that teaching psychiatrists psychotherapy helps them become better caregivers for their patients; that this training mandate, when understood in the context of a broader move toward eclecticism in psychiatry, can be construed as a strategy for defending against increasingly common jurisdictional incursions; and, finally, that psychiatrists who are at least conversant in nonpharmacological treatments can help bridge divisions in the field of mental health.

IMPLICATIONS FOR PSYCHIATRY RESIDENTS' TRAINING AND PROFESSIONAL IDENTITIES

A Shorewood graduate once told me that "psychiatrists can't afford to say that they don't know anything about therapy." Indeed, partly because their pharmacological tools have fallen short of offering cures and partly because they work in a field divided among epistemic communities, psychiatrists must have at least a modicum of familiarity with, if not also competence in, the main alternative to pharmacology; namely, psychotherapy. But what this means for the residents' training and for their professional identities is a matter of debate.

Although the psychiatry residents I spent time with eventually did develop psychotherapeutic competencies and came to see the value of training in these approaches, they did not always agree on how much of their schedules should be taken up by the process. Disagreements centered on psychodynamic training, as it took up more of the residents' time than other approaches. Gordon, a senior resident (PGY-4), believed that psychodynamic training ought to be a "bigger priority for residents," with "more protected" time dedicated to it. "I would hate to add more, you know, to the [residents'] schedule," Gordon explained, "but I think there's a way to do that where it's not stressful for the resident." Vinit (PGY-4) told his colleagues and instructors that "seeing your first psychodynamic patient in the end of PGY-2 year [second postgraduate year] and beginning of PGY-3 year [third postgraduate year] is unfortunate," because, he stressed, "you miss out on a lot. I think it should be forced upon us." His surprising choice of words was telling: though the residents started out skeptical about the time they dedicated to psychotherapy, some ended up thinking that they needed more of it.[17] Not all the residents felt this way.

Sawyer (PGY-4) concurred with his colleague's assessment of "the value" of learning psychodynamic psychotherapy but thought that the residents already dedicated many hours to the "psychodynamic experience." He added, "Augmenting it makes me nervous. What I would be enthusiastic about is making it more efficient." These disagreements reflected the concern of many psychiatrists involved in residency education: how should trainees' time be split up to ensure that the field produces well-rounded professionals who can become experts in neurobiology while also engaging competently with other interventions?

But the residents' disagreements about how to apportion their training time hinted at a deeper question. Their concerns were fundamentally about what makes a good psychiatrist. In this context, Dr. Jackson, the Shorewood residency director, was right to ask (rhetorically), "Why bother doing therapy training when most people don't end up actually doing therapy when they get out of here?" And, among the therapies, why have "analytic training" at all? Psychiatry residents, I was repeatedly told, would not learn enough therapy to become therapists. This was not a return to the psychiatry of the 1950s, '60s, and '70s. Instead, the thinking went, as they learned psychotherapy, particularly the psychodynamic type, the residents would improve their skills in relating to and treating their patients.

I came to agree with Dr. Jackson, who, after speaking technically and at length about residency requirements and the challenges of implementing them, told me that the residents become "better doctors" because of therapeutic training. Compared with earlier residents who did not benefit from such training, those learning psychotherapy were less "mechanistic" in their work, as one of the Shorewood instructors put it. They came to view their roles as not simply mending diseased brains but as caring for people.[18]

This shift depended on developing flexible doctoring repertoires that included not only pharmacological tools but also talk and behavioral ones. Psychotherapy prepared the residents to become the kind of doctors who could recognize when a medication prescription was indicated, or when a patient could weather a crisis with the help of a CBT technique, or when their request for an increased medication dosage was in fact motivated by difficult life circumstances. Psychiatrists' familiarity with psychotherapy could thus facilitate better patient care because they could appeal to distinct explanations for their patients' suffering and to appropriate treatments to ease it.

Indeed, this is precisely what the residents at Shorewood were able to do as they became competent in psychotherapy. Most found some of the psychotherapeutic approaches they learned compelling enough to pragmatically accommodate them within their existing doctoring repertoires.

A minority went on to practice psychotherapy and dedicated themselves to honing their hybrid repertoires through further psychotherapy training.[19] This should not be taken to mean that any of these psychiatrists had an easy path toward integrating biological and talk therapeutic approaches. Rather, they had to carve out their own space in a field set up to maintain just such divisions.

But, whether or not they would go on to practice psychotherapy, these doctors were better prepared to help patients when medications were insufficient or even unnecessary. Arguably, one of the biggest payoffs of psychotherapeutic training in psychiatry is that it prepares biopsychiatrists to act when their pharmacological tools fall short. Learning to recognize the constellation of factors that may make a patient's condition more amenable to CBT or psychodynamic treatment—in addition to or instead of psychiatric medications—is a valuable skill. Rather than deeming patients who see few, if any, benefits from chemical interventions "treatment resistant," psychiatrists who are conversant in psychotherapy can, at a minimum, direct such patients to specialists in alternative treatments.[20]

IMPLICATIONS FOR THE PROFESSION OF PSYCHIATRY

An eclectic epistemic tool kit may also be the key to psychiatry's continued jurisdictional power. As mental illness has continued to elude psychiatrists' grasp, uncertainty—or even, as sociologist Owen Whooley has proposed, "ignorance"—has become their profession's persistent and defining state.[21] The story that this book tells can thus also be read as a story about how psychiatrists negotiate this broader uncertainty while struggling to remain dominant in the field of mental health. Put simply, psychotherapy training in psychiatry—when viewed as part of a larger turn toward eclecticism— can be seen as a professional strategy for warding off jurisdictional threats, even if only temporarily.

The psychiatric profession's dominance has long rested on shifting ground. Writing about psychiatry in the 1980s, sociologist Andrew Abbott proposed that its strength was due to the coherence offered by psychoanalytic theories.[22] Yet this power vanished during that same decade, replaced by the rapid rise of pharmacology. This, too, seemed to solve psychiatry's professional and epistemic problems, at least for a while. Nevertheless, despite its successful campaign to render mental suffering biological, and a "decade of the brain" that brought much federal investment in neuroscientific research, the search for the biological mechanisms and cures of mental illness has remained inconclusive.

Making matters more precarious, contemporary psychiatry has been facing jurisdictional incursions from inside and outside the field of mental health. According to a 2009 study, primary care physicians account for 59 percent of psychiatric drug prescriptions, leading in antianxiety medications, antidepressants, and stimulants.[23] Psychologists, too, have begun to encroach on psychiatrists' prescribing privileges, scoring significant victories in six US states where they can now manage psychopharmaceuticals alongside psychiatrists, psychiatric nurse practitioners, and family doctors.[24]

On their own, these trends give the impression of an overdetermined future, one in which the psychiatric profession will eventually be rendered obsolete. Yet psychiatrists retain leading positions in the field, evidenced by their roles in crafting the much critiqued but still essential *Diagnostic and Statistical Manual of Mental Disorders*, leading research teams, and setting the practice guidelines for prescribing psychotropic medications that all other health care professionals rely on. Moreover, since 2011, the number of graduating medical students who choose to specialize in psychiatry—and the number of psychiatric residencies training them—has steadily grown.[25] This suggests a more complicated view of the profession's future. Nevertheless, with drugs no longer under their exclusive control, psychiatrists are needing and finding new ways to safeguard their domain.

An eclectic repertoire may help the profession fend off, at least for a time, jurisdictional threats. Along with a recommitment to psychotherapy, the twenty-first century has seen psychiatry return to electroconvulsive therapy and other brain stimulation techniques, while also rediscovering a variety of psychedelic treatments. All the while, the profession has redoubled its commitments to neuroscience and to research into the genetic roots of mental illness. The profession is expanding its repertoire to include a wider range of approaches, even as its clinicians remain, by and large, focused on the pharmaceutical management of mental illness.[26]

To some in the field, this eclecticism is a positive reflection of the "biopsychosocial" model of care.[27] In a 2022 editorial published in the *American Journal of Psychiatry*, Dr. Ned Kalin, a psychiatrist at the University of Wisconsin's School of Medicine, proposed that "psychiatry, perhaps more than any other discipline in medicine, has embraced the integrated use of complementary psychosocial and biological interventions."[28] For proponents of the biopsychosocial approach, psychotherapeutic training offers an important corrective to the reductionism of biological perspectives.[29] For example, Glen Gabbard and Jerald Kay, two psychiatrists who have written extensively about the value of psychotherapy, have argued that the "biopsychosocial model is crucial in every clinical setting."[30] Not only is combining psychotherapy and medications best for patients, they argue, but psychotherapy can also enhance patients' adherence to pharmacological regimens. Significantly, these psychiatrists propose, "the unique capacity to conduct integrated treatment" is what sets their profession apart from other mental health practitioners and from other physicians alike.[31] Put simply, when properly enacted, the biopsychosocial approach can strengthen psychiatrists' position in the field of mental health and medicine more broadly, assuring their professional standing. Competence in psychotherapy can get psychiatrists closer to this goal.

But these perspectives of an "integrated" model of care appear divorced from how most psychiatrists work. Increased specialization means that today, the biopsychosocial model of care has remained dispersed across specializations, such that, by and large, psychiatrists deal with biology, psychologists with psychology, and social workers with patients' social needs. Yet psychiatrists cannot fully ignore the psychological and social dimensions of their patients' suffering even if they themselves do not offer solutions in these domains. After all, as the residents knew well, drugs do not always work. Moreover, psychiatrists continue to work alongside psychologists and social workers as they care for patients in clinics and hospitals. Being at least conversant, if not also competent, in psychotherapy, the most commonly used alternative to pharmacology, enables them to act as more informed coordinators of patient care and leaders of multi-professional teams.

IMPLICATIONS FOR THE BROADER FIELD OF MENTAL HEALTH

One of the key takeaways of the analysis in this book is that the productive management of skepticism is central to the resilience of fields that are, like mental health, divided among epistemic communities. Psychiatrists, psychologists, and social workers have their own training institutions and requirements, and their own professional associations.[32] Further divisions are instituted in approach-specific societies that sometimes cross professional boundaries.[33] Each of these societies, in turn, has its own vision of what causes mental illness and how to best treat it. But, in a context where the goal is to maintain a professional arrangement that "keeps everybody in business," as one of the residents put it, psychiatrists' shift toward psychotherapy may run contrary to the interests of other professionals in the field. In fact, "hybrids," sociologist Gil Eyal has argued, can be threatening to an existing order organized around boundaries between occupational domains.[34]

However, there are powerful countervailing forces that disincentivize psychiatrists from fully adopting hybrid repertoires of action and encroaching on other professionals' psychotherapeutic domains. The experiences of residents who tried to put their psychotherapeutic commitments into practice are telling in this respect. Those who wanted to translate their hybrid repertoires into more durable professional paths—by, for example, seeking jobs that would allow them to prescribe and also do talk therapy with their patients—encountered a system that is set up to expel them.[35] Insurers do not reimburse psychotherapy at the same rate as they do medication appointments. Nor do they readily pay for it when it is delivered by the most expensive member of the mental health field: a psychiatrist. This means that a formal commitment to doing psychotherapy with one's patients entails real economic sacrifices for psychiatrists. They must set aside time in their schedules for forty-five-minute psychotherapy appointments and forgo the material benefits of seeing three patients for fifteen-minute medication management sessions during that same period. This is as an important structural barrier to psychiatrists who may wish to do therapy but must also pay back student loans while building adult lives. Along with their biopsychiatric socialization, these material concerns may help explain why so few psychiatrists pursue hybrid professional paths. The only alternative—and the one that dominates the professional landscape today—is that psychiatrists stick to pharmacology, while psychologists and social workers take on the psychological and social dimensions of patients' illnesses.

Nevertheless, biopsychiatrists who are also conversant in psychotherapy can serve an important bridging role between epistemic and professional communities. They can act as well-informed referral nodes, steering patients toward other appropriately trained mental health professionals. They can facilitate the kind of collaboration deemed essential to effective research and care in the field of mental health. Finally, they can help find solutions when conflicting perspectives dispose their colleagues toward disagreement over how to make sense of a patient's suffering or course of treatment.

Such integrative work depends, however, on access to institutional contexts conducive to cooperation. Training programs, clinics, and other spaces where diverse professionals can engage with one another play key roles in the collective management of skepticism. Whether in training rotations, case consultations, or group supervision, psychiatrists and other mental health practitioners can question their assumptions, exchange ideas, and coordinate action.[36] The psychotherapy meetings that the residents participated in are examples of just such spaces of cross-professional exchange. Here, psychotherapists (instructors, supervisors, and, in some cases, trainees) and psychiatrists (the residents) came together with the manifest purpose of training and education. But with each patient whose problems came up for discussion, biopsychiatrists and psychotherapists collaborated to develop workable interventions, crossing epistemic and professional boundaries. These clinical and instructional spaces were thus as much about learning as they were about collectively working through and toward epistemic and professional accommodation.

Implications for Research on Work and Occupations

This book's theoretical scaffolding is built on the scholarship on professions, work, and expertise. But, because of psychiatry's particularities, we might assume that the kind of frictions and skepticism the previous pages have outlined are unique to it. Nevertheless, instead of pursuing empirical generalization, I propose that the theoretical mechanisms I have elaborated can be fruitfully employed to understand the conundrums of professionals in other contexts.[37] Contradictory roles marked by epistemic and professional friction abound. Medical professionals have had to confront reforms that challenged their understandings of their core tasks and professional identities.[38] In academia, interdisciplinarity has become increasingly dominant, premised on the assumption that crossing disciplinary boundaries can solve common problems.[39] But organizational and epistemic changes that compel professionals to work across domains is laden with challenges, especially when they sense threats to their own expertise and jurisdiction.[40] Put simply, whether spurred by reform or by the structure of the task, friction is constitutive of professional expert work.

Extant scholarship has framed such friction in terms of jurisdictional conflicts revolving around symbolic or material boundary drawing.[41] In contrast, sociologist Gil Eyal has proposed that, to understand how a task is accomplished, we must attend to the "arrangements" or "networks" that link various actors, materials, and social relations necessary for its completion. Whereas the jurisdictional perspective has focused on professional struggles, the relational one has largely overlooked them. This book has proposed that although jurisdictional conflict is at times a concern for professionals, it is not always the overriding driver of action. Instead, professionals are, by and large, oriented toward solving problems and accomplishing tasks in line with their envisioned identities. And while relational work is constitutive of this process, it is not itself frictionless. Attending to such frictions is paramount if we are to understand how professionals participate in "networks of expertise," to borrow Eyal's phrase, that involve differently positioned human and nonhuman actors.[42]

More important, this book calls for greater attention to the dynamics of skepticism and its collective management in professional settings. The inevitable corollary to friction, skepticism is a stance that can be defensive and productive in particular social and institutional conditions. To be sure, skepticism need not always find its resolution in the development of new competencies and new knowledge. But, whatever its resolution, skepticism is a feature of expert groups and their practices, whether it serves as a tool of professional control, a stance that needs managing to establish credibility and enable innovation, or an inherent part of generating new knowledge.[43] The previous pages have offered an integrated and dynamic theory of skepticism by showing how it stems from conditions of friction, how contexts set up for validation, observation, and experimentation can help in its management, and how skepticism can give way to self-reflexivity and, eventually, expanded professional repertoires. Friction and skepticism, in other words, are constitutive of processes of change and interprofessional collaboration and require ongoing practical management.

Broader shifts in the landscape of professionalism are making these considerations relevant in new ways. Scholars have shown that, since the 1990s, workers have become increasingly committed to their professional identities rather than their employers, with the percentage of people who work on a "contract" basis having steadily grown.[44] This trend toward contract work, however, necessitates the flexibility to navigate new organizational domains and even learn new skills, as the job demands. This shift is connected to a second development, one that organizational scholars Herminia Ibarra and Otilia Obodaru have described as the proliferation of "liminality" in contemporary careers.[45] As workers become agents of their employment—seeking out the next contract, client, or opportunity—they find themselves in a persistent state of transition. Pivoting between jobs, gigs, or projects forces contemporary professionals to continuously adjust to new organizational or epistemic demands, navigating frictions between their existing skills and the new ones they must learn, between being insiders and outsiders. Studying how professionals adopt, modify, or reject these ever-present sources of friction can help scholars of work and occupations map how being in persistent flux affects contemporary workers' identities and expert repertoires.

This book suggests that, to grasp how professionals achieve self-sufficiency and self-efficacy in conditions that are rife with contradictions, we must attend to the dynamics of friction and skepticism and the relational conditions that facilitate their resolution. The book's central argument has been that professional and epistemic friction constitute fertile ground for skepticism, a stance that allows people to establish their worth in conditions that seem structured to undermine it. Left unaddressed, such doubts can become a hardened shell that precludes more flexible engagements with new professional or epistemic demands. However, relational contexts in which professionals receive recognition for their struggles, witness new forms of expertise in action, and get to experiment with new skills and roles in relatively low-stakes situations can render skepticism productive, enabling change. Skepticism's management, in turn, is a collective undertaking that depends on trusted interlocutors and that, in turn, constitutes professionals, their repertoires of action, and their identities.

ACKNOWLEDGMENTS

This book has been a long time in the making. It—and I—have benefited from the support of many people and institutions. First, none of this would have been possible were it not for the generosity of Shorewood educators and trainees. Though I am unable to thank them by name, I am grateful that they welcomed me into their conference rooms, offices, and, sometimes, homes, tolerating my frequently ignorant questions and sharing with me parts of their lives. The fundamental lesson they taught me is the importance of approaching others with curiosity and compassion—a worthy pursuit for ethnographers and psychiatrists alike. I hope that the book reflects a slice of their worlds and offers something instructive in return.

Research for the book started during my graduate work, and I benefited immensely from the guidance and support of my doctoral committee: Jason Owen-Smith, Renee Anspach, Geneviève Zubrzycki, George Steinmetz, and John Carson. Jason has been an extraordinary mentor since my first year at the University of Michigan, reading endless drafts of papers, chapters, and grant applications, sending out a never-ending stream of letters of recommendation, and offering me advice on topics ranging from research to the job market and life with a family. His ongoing encouragement and counsel are my lifelines in academia. Renee Anspach has been an engaged and patient interlocutor, helping to clarify my thinking about psychotherapy and serving as my insightful and forgiving guide through the scholarship on professions and medicine. I met Geneviève Zubrzycki as a prospective student during my visit to Ann Arbor, and I have her to thank for helping me through some of the best and most significant decisions I've made since, both intellectual and personal. George Steinmetz impressed upon me the import of what we do as sociologists and the fact that big ideas are not meant to be venerated but, rather, questioned and engaged with. John Carson did not know me before I asked whether he would serve on my doctoral committee, but he took to the task with enthusiasm, decidedly improving both my work and my professional life. Together, these five extraordinary scholars not only shaped my thinking but also embodied the generosity, thoughtfulness, and reasonableness that I assumed only belonged in descriptions of academic ideal types. Most importantly, they showed me that I too could be part of this profession.

This book lived its first life at Northwestern University, where I held a postdoctoral position in the Science in Human Culture (SHC) Program and the Sociology Department. I am especially grateful to Steve Epstein, my mentor, for helping me in many ways, including thinking through the book when it was still in its embryonic stages. Along with Héctor Carrillo, he helped make Northwestern into a welcoming and intellectually vibrant academic home. Chas Camic and Beth Mertz were incredibly supportive and generous. I very much miss our ice cream dates and their gentle guidance. Carol Heimer, Tony Chen, Christine Percheski, Ann Orloff, Wendy Espeland, Laura Beth Nielsen, and Bob Nelson helped me find my place in the Sociology Department. At SHC, I am grateful to Ken Alder and Helen Tilley for fostering such an energetic, engaged, and open community. Paul Ramirez, Rebecca Seligman, Daniel Immerwahr, and Laura Pedraza Farina offered both intellectual stimulation and an empathic ear on topics ranging from research and writing to the job market. During my time at SHC, I was lucky to overlap with an outstanding group of postdoctoral fellows that included Tania Munz, Daniel Stolz, Aaron Norton, Stefanie Graeter, and Fredrik Meiton. Tania changed my life (with Leo) and stoked my confidence. Dan showed me that patience eventually pays off.

More friends, colleagues, and mentors played pivotal roles as the book began to take shape. Camilo Arturo Leslie and Kim Greenwell have lived with this project as long as I have. They both read more versions of chapters than they (and I) wish to remember, soothed tense nerves as frequently as was necessary, and repeatedly reminded me that I could get this done. Camilo became an expert at late-evening conversations as I grumpily and urgently struggled with ideas big and small. Kim has mastered the editorial arts, knowing exactly what kind of advice I needed when and, most importantly, always coming up with practical solutions to my thorniest problems. Stefan Timmermans has generously and brilliantly helped this project along even before he took it on as editor of the Ethnographic Encounters and Discoveries series at the University of Chicago Press. His constructive comments and questions always had the effect of clarifying and sharpening my thinking and writing. I hope the book now delivers on his much-prized triumvirate: a hook, an arc, and good writing. Owen Whooley approached my ideas and writing with curiosity and a readiness to help. His pages and pages of detailed comments on an earlier version of the manuscript and his suggestion that I read Charles Peirce's writing on doubt were crucial in shaping the final draft. Andy McDowell has been my writing partner through much of this book's life. Our conversations kept me inspired, our deadlines kept me writing, and our commiseration kept me sane.

Others have also offered much-needed encouragement, comments, and thoughtfulness along the way. Charles Bosk (d. 2020) extended me warm welcome and gave me more sage advice than I could successfully imprint into memory. I wish he could have seen the book done—I'm sure I would have had much to learn from his responses. Gil Eyal has been a brilliant and extremely generous interlocutor on the topics of therapy and expertise. Tania Jenkins and Dan Menchik have offered advice on the sociology of professions and on how to be a professional sociologist. Claudio Benzecry helped me work through a thorny question about the book's arc. Claire Decoteau always lent a wise ear and inspired by example. Laura Hirshfield and the core members of the HPE group have been a consistent source of inspiration and support. At Tulane, David Smilde and Katie Johnson read an early version of the manuscript and offered insightful comments. My colleagues Mimi Schippers, Michele Adams, and Patrick Rafail have encouraged me along the way. Robin Bartram offered great company, practical advice, and support. I feel especially lucky to have Amalia Leguizamón as a colleague and a friend—she's made being here infinitely better. Maria Farkas, Claire Decoteau and Andy Clarno, Jothie Rajah, Susan Shapiro, Meredith Rountree and Rob Owen, Subah Dayal and Tyson Patros, Cheryl Naruse and Steven Gin, and Molly Pulda and Gary Sernovitz have offered wise words and nourishment of all kinds.

Various institutions supported the research and writing process. At the University of Michigan, grants from the Center for the Education of Women and the Rackham Graduate School enabled me to complete my doctoral work. Northwestern University funded my travel to various research sites. The National Science Foundation helped me extend my postdoctoral position and make progress on what I thought would be my first book but is now turning out to be my next project. At Tulane, grants from the Office of the Provost, the Carol Lavin Bernick program, the Louisiana Board of Regents Awards to Louisiana Artists and Scholars Program (ATLAS), and the School of Liberal Arts allowed me to connect with mentors, hold a book-manuscript workshop, and make progress on revisions.

At the University of Chicago Press, Elizabeth Branch Dyson has steadily guided me toward the finish line and was the first to suggest skepticism as the book's organizing theme (I was characteristically skeptical of her suggestion!). Mollie McFee has offered expert and timely assistance and was the one to remind me that the book *will* be published. Stephen Twilley has been my generous guide through the production process. The marketing and cover design teams have done outstanding work. I am grateful also to my careful copy editor, Lori Meek Schuldt, and my indexer, Lisa DeBoer. Finally, I am thankful to the reviewers for offering extremely helpful insights early in the process.

Usually, families remain behind the scenes doing the hard but taken-for-granted work of keeping authors fed and healthy, sane and human. Mine did all that and more. My parents, Eugenia Crăciun and Gheorghe Crăciun, made the fateful decision to move our family to the United States from Romania, cutting short my dreams of traveling the world as a translator and inadvertently putting me on a path toward sociology. Without my parents' courage, patience, and absolute belief in the power of learning, this book would have never happened. My sisters, Florentina and Claudia Crăciun, have offered both support and diversion. They asked about my work, celebrated my successes, and always kept up the excitement of being part of our family. Nowadays, they do so alongside their husbands, Sean Cannon and Burgess Tomlinson; they have made my life better by making my sisters happy. Dora Tomlinson, my sweet niece, makes me smile with her high jinks. My cousin, Geanina Alina Ionescu, always saw more in me than I could. Her love and belief in my capacities continue to sustain me along all of life's ways.

My deepest gratitude goes to Camilo, Eva, and Sally. Camilo's brilliance, his sense of humor, his stores upon stores of patience, his knowledge of (almost) all things, and his resolute faith in my ability to get things done have helped me be both a person and an academic. Sally has been our incredibly sweet and gentle companion, infusing our lives with love, calm, and unconditional acceptance (though there are lots of treats, too!). I can't imagine a day at my office without her. Eva made the process of writing this book infinitely more joyful. Herself an avid reader, she was shocked to learn that both her parents are writing books, and even more shocked that they don't have any pictures. After a brief period of disappointment, she became an insightful inquirer about what we do. Her curiosity, creativity, smarts, silliness, determination, and overall effervescence never cease to amaze me. Together, Camilo, Eva, and Sally have made possible a life I could not have imagined. This book is for them.

Appendix

I did not set out to study skepticism, but it was part of my research all along. I started this project hoping to learn about therapeutic expertise: what therapists did, how they thought about their patients' problems, how they felt, and whether they could stop being therapists when they walked out of their offices at the end of the day. I was particularly interested in comparing what it meant to be a therapist in the psychoanalytic tradition and the so-called evidence-based approaches, cognitive behavioral therapy (CBT) dominant among them. Observing novices learning psychotherapy was thus part of a larger project that eventually included interviews with sixty psychotherapists, some in each epistemic community.

Though I had not initially thought of Shorewood as my primary field site, a series of access denials turned it into my main locus of observations. The process of gaining access began to reveal the role of skepticism in the mental health professions. As I sought to secure entry into a site, I was given the opportunity to present my research at one psychoanalytic institute and at Shorewood. The conversations I had in the process were illuminating. Confidentiality was a principal concern: patients' stories would be discussed in the meetings I would be sitting in on, and patients themselves may, from time to time, be present in such settings, and I was not a trained medical professional. I had, however, received training in the ethics of qualitative research and in protecting human subjects, both at the Institutional Review Board and later when I joined the clinic. To protect patients, I followed common ethical practices in the field of mental health and in my own discipline of sociology.

The mental health professionals I spent time with were themselves sensitive to issues of confidentiality. They protected their own patients by sharing very little identifying information when they discussed their treatments; this, in turn, made my job easier, as there was less I needed to conceal in my own notes. Moreover, akin to the practitioners I spent time with, I was prepared to leave the room if anyone I was familiar with ever came up for discussion in the groups. That never happened, though at one point a resident had to leave because the patient whose case was being discussed was a friend of an acquaintance. While taking notes, I myself was mindful of what made it into in my files. When bits of information about a patient, such as the name of their neighborhood or locality, or place of employment, did show up in conversation, I did not record them. Nor did I write down details about the patient's illness experience that were so unique that someone could easily identify them. Lastly, when I did find myself in the same room with patients, I was introduced as part of the group, and I followed the example of the other participants, adopting an appropriate affective demeanor as well as taking only minimal notes about the exchanges so as not to disturb the proceedings.

Patients, however, were not the only subjects of concern. I was seeking entry into a world where becoming professional has as much to do with attending to patients' inner lives as it does with shaping one's own. When I met with the members of a committee running one of the local psychoanalytic organizations, the issue became clearer. Here are some notes I took afterward:

> At yesterday's committee meeting I gave a brief presentation of my project and answered questions. I did a good job (I think) of allaying their fears about patient confidentiality, but a different issue emerged. [One of the psychoanalytic supervisors] was the one who named it, and he had also brought it up in our previous [one-on-one] meeting in September. The issue is that of the vulnerability that therapists experience in these classes when discussing cases. This, he argued, is because they end up disclosing much of themselves, and the presence of an outsider may endanger/change the dynamics in the room. To address this issue, I will be meeting with the [psychoanalytic] candidates this coming Sunday.

To help patients make sense of and manage their inner lives, novices had to learn to discipline their own. This learning process, as I have shown throughout the book, took place in conversations: with peers, with instructors and supervisors, with other members of the therapeutic community. Allowing me to observe some of these discussions, particularly those of a more intimate nature, could distort the process. Eventually, I did speak to the psychoanalytic candidates and, though they did have some concerns about this issue, they ultimately approved my request.

Yet my conversation with the candidates also made me aware of another, thornier, issue. When I explained that I was interested in comparing psychodynamic and CBT forms of expertise, the psychoanalysts-in-training stressed the benefits and advantages of their own approach. But one of the participants found her colleagues' declarations needlessly defensive and chastised them for "revealing their insecurities with regards to CBT." Becoming a psychoanalyst was a formidable choice in an epistemic and institutional context that seemed to favor the faster and seemingly more effective cognitive and behavioral interventions. The psychoanalytic candidates and supervisors were weary of a sociologist coming into their midst and possibly uncovering their "insecurities."

Feeling under threat was not, however, the sole territory of psychoanalysts. One Shorewood affiliate told me that he was happy I was going to observe CBT rotations because "evidence-based therapies" had been "marginalized." My fieldwork, he believed, would help undo some of the doubts he had himself encountered, thus helping to legitimate this work. I was surprised to hear such an assertion, given my understanding that CBT and related approaches were dominant among psychotherapies at the time. I would later come to understand these concerns as valid in the context of CBT's relatively marginal position in psychiatry itself. Psychiatry has had a long, if also turbulent, relationship with psychoanalysis. In this context, CBT was still the newcomer, seeking to establish its bona fides to a profession that seemed disposed against it. For the residents however, CBT's affinities with biopsychiatry proved a boon, easing their entry into the unfamiliar world of doctoring without drugs.

Nevertheless, these conversations revealed that the work of legitimation I would later observe instructors do at Shorewood was already taking place in my earliest encounters in the field. And while some instructors hoped I would help them with their cause, others were more skeptical of my aims. After one such meeting, I wrote in my research notebook: *There seems to be a great deal of suspicion about what I will do with my data and who will have access to it.* After another meeting, I added: *The people I want to observe are worried about being evaluated; they want to know how I will use my findings.* I then realized that I had to address a key question that loomed over my project. I had to explain to my interlocutors that, in fact, I was not planning on—nor was I equipped to—compare the effectiveness of psychodynamic and cognitive behavioral interventions. I was simply looking to learn more about what it meant to be an expert in these approaches.

Finally, and unbeknownst to me at the time, I had asked for permission to observe the residents' psychotherapy training at a time when Shorewood was expanding its therapeutic offerings and new instructors were joining the program. Worries about evaluation or about who will have access to my data were thus not fueled simply by concerns that I would compare different therapeutic approaches but also by apprehension about assessing these ongoing efforts and the instructors' own competence. As soon as I caught onto this new source of doubt, I quickly addressed it by assuring the instructors that I had no such intention. I hope also that my book convinces the reader that, no matter how masterly an instructor, they had considerable odds to overcome when training psychiatry residents. After all, they had little control over the residents' earlier socialization in biopsychiatry or their expectations about their professional trajectories.

After I secured buy-in from the experienced clinicians who served as the residents' instructors at Shorewood, two hurdles remained: gaining the approval of the residency education director and that of the residents themselves. I worried about facing the director, as my track record had not been altogether successful when it came to the higher ranks of the institutions I had approached for field access. At this point, months into my efforts to gain entry into an ethnographic field site, I was prepared for rejection. Yet my meeting with Dr. Jackson went surprisingly well. He had read T. M. Luhrmann's ethnography of psychiatric training, *Of Two Minds*, and imagined I would do something similar. Though that was not quite my intent (my project was narrower in scope with respect to the residents' education), I appreciated Dr. Jackson's familiarity with the kind of work I was proposing and felt grateful to Luhrmann for paving the way through her book. Soon thereafter, Dr. Jackson wrote an email to the residents informing them that I would join their psychotherapy rotations.

The residents, too, were very open to my efforts. I introduced myself and the general outlines of my project at the beginning of every rotation and explained that, though Dr. Jackson had given me his approval, the residents were free to choose to not be part of my research. I negotiated access in this manner regularly with each entry into a new training setting and each new participant in the rotations. Just once did an invited psychotherapist decline participation, only to conclude at the end of the meeting that it would have been all right for me to take notes on the discussion after all. Throughout, the residents themselves were welcoming and offered to help as best they could. When the situation permitted, they instructed me on the goings-on of the discussion or on the differential uses of pharmaceuticals or psychotherapy.

After I received IRB approval and began my observations at Shorewood and at the local psychoanalytic institute, it became evident that Shorewood would be sufficiently productive for my research purposes. Conversations at Shorewood were clinically oriented and practical, whereas those at the institute were, unsurprisingly, focused on psychoanalytic theories and ideas, with the occasional reference to work with patients. More interesting for me, discussions at Shorewood quickly hinted at broader tensions in the field of mental health: between biopsychiatry and psychotherapy, between particular psychotherapeutic approaches and their devotees, and between residents and psychotherapy instructors and supervisors.

What I did not take notice of analytically right away was the skepticism that the particular novices I observed—the psychiatry residents—brought to the process of learning psychotherapy. Though I had been met with doubt when I sought research access, the residents' own doubts were less evident to me. Nevertheless, as I became more attuned to the residents' skepticism, I came to also understand the contradictions that characterized their positions. Finally, I also came to appreciate the skepticism that others—whether psychoanalysts, CBT clinicians, trainees, supervisors, or instructors—aimed at my project. With time, I understood it as more than the typical barriers that autonomous professionals construct in the face of curious interlopers. Rather, in expressing their doubts, the professionals revealed the unsettledness of the field itself and the struggles that its members undertook in their search for legitimacy. And while we might assume that such doubts would undo the field of mental health, in fact, as I argue in the concluding chapter of the book, I came to think of skepticism and its collective management as constitutive of the field itself.

NOTES

Chapter One

1. Grinker 1964, 228.

2. Klitzman 1995, 37.

3. Lieberman and Ogas 2015, 69. Dr. Lieberman was paraphrasing and elaborating Sigmund Freud's reported remark to Carl Jung upon their 1909 arrival in the United States, where Freud delivered his only address to an American audience at Clark University (Lieberman and Ogas 2015, 64).

4. Lieberman and Ogas 2015, quotations at 292, 10 (italics in original).

5. For other examples of how contemporary psychiatrists describe their profession's changes, see Harrington 2019, xi–xiii, Metzl 2003, 1–4; Whooley 2019, 117–28.

6. Insel 2022, 103–8.

7. Insel 2022, 51–52, 101–3; Lieberman and Ogas 2015, 224–29.

8. Detre and McDonald 1997, 203.

9. This and all other names associated with research participants are pseudonyms.

10. Borderline personality disorder is characterized by intense fear of abandonment, unstable relationships, anger, and impulsive behaviors (for full list of criteria, see American Psychiatric Association 2013).

11. PGY stands for *postgraduate year*, and it refers to residency years following medical school. It is a common way of indicating a doctor's year in residency, e.g., PGY-4 corresponds to a fourth-year resident.

12. Other scholars have appealed to friction to describe global connections (Tsing 2005), oppression and resistance (Medina 2013), and knowledge and truth (Sher 2016). Anthropologist Anna Lowenhaupt Tsing argued for sustained attention to "cross-culture and long-distance encounters in forming everything we know as culture" (Tsing 2005, 4). Such "interconnections across difference" (Tsing 2005, 4) are generative of misunderstanding and friction but can also produce alliances. For their part, science and technology scholars have long—if largely implicitly—attended to friction: between science and nonscience (e.g., Gieryn 1983, 1999), fact and artifact (e.g., Latour 1987; Latour and Woolgar 1979), lay and expert (e.g. Epstein 1996, 1997), field and laboratory (e.g. Gieryn 2006; Knorr Cetina 1992). What emerges in these studies is the instability of such demarcations, as credibility and expertise are persistently contested and negotiated.

13. Sadowsky 2006, 6.

14. Historical accounts of the emergence and initial uptake of psychopharmaceuticals include Harrington 2019; Healy 1997, 2002; Herzberg 2009; Horwitz 2002; Metzl 2003; Sadowsky 2021; Whooley 2019.

15. Abbott 1988.

16. When the NIMH was founded in 1949, it was tasked not only with supporting the training of psychiatrists but also with answering questions about which treatments worked and why. Early on, it channeled some of its resources into researching how psychoanalysis helped patients and what made some practitioners more effective than others. But when these inquiries failed to generate significant breakthroughs, the agency turned its support toward biological research, controlled randomized clinical trials (RCTs), and epidemiological studies. For NIMH and psychotherapy research and training, see, e.g., Parloff and Elkin 1992; Pickren and Schneider 2005. For a history of the Menninger brothers' influence and research, see Hale 1995.

17. In this framework, a psychiatric drug could help with symptom management and make patients more amenable to psychoanalysis. See, e.g., Healy 1997; Herzberg 2009; Metzl 2003; Sadowsky 2021.

18. Hale 1995, 248. Ethnographies of psychiatry residencies during the latter years of psychoanalytic dominance include work by Coser (1979) and Light (1980); for an earlier look at psychiatric work, including how residents trained, see Strauss et al. 1964.

19. See, e.g., Hale 1995; Grob 1994; Mechanic 2008.

20. On deinstitutionalization, see, e.g., Grob 1994; Whooley 2019.

21. See, e.g., T. Mark et al. 2018; D. Smith 2019; West et al. 2003; Wilk et al. 2006.

22. Feighner et al. 1972.

23. Feighner et al. 1972, 57.

24. The diagnostic standards that the St. Louis group outlined, later known as the Feighner criteria, played a pivotal role in the DSM-III. Robert Spitzer, the psychiatrist who led the revision efforts, granted the group and other like-minded psychiatrist-researchers prominent roles in the process. Their aim was to devise an "atheoretical" diagnostic system that focused on the observable behaviors associated with particular illnesses. This was a radical departure from psychoanalysts' explicitly theoretical search for the causes of mental illness. Nevertheless, though it was hailed as a "paradigm shift" by its proponents, the published version of the manual ended up accommodating both perspectives. The DSM-III was organized around multiple axes that included common mental conditions such as major depression and anxiety on Axis I—reflecting the research emphasis of the St. Louis group—as well as the personality disorders on Axis II that had been psychoanalysts' primary foci. The revised DSM had wide-ranging implications for patients, practitioners, and organizations. The new psychiatric diagnoses reduced the psychoanalytic complexity of mental illness and systematized the process of identifying it. They were essential for standardizing illness identities, insurance reimbursements, and drug development (in sociological terms, the DSM-III achieved what Lakoff [2005a] called "diagnostic liquidity"). But the DSM-III's publication also had unanticipated and troubling consequences. The manual proved especially productive for pharmaceutical companies as they capitalized on the relatively flexible boundaries of the diagnostic categories it codified. Beginning in the 1970s, pharmaceutical companies redoubled their efforts at finding new psychotropics and obtaining the approval of the Food and Drug Administration (FDA) to bring them to market. Aided by the legalization of direct-to-consumer-advertising in 1997,

pharmaceutical companies could brand not only drugs but also psychiatric diagnoses themselves, turning everyday shyness or sadness into mental disorders. This practice resulted in billions of dollars in profit from the sales of Prozac, Paxil, and Zoloft, to name just some of the blockbuster psychotropic medications. Literature on the DSM and its revisions, as well as its role in transforming the profession of psychiatry, is extensive. Standout social scientific accounts include Kirk and Kutchins 1992 as well as Harrington 2019; Herzberg 2009; Horwitz 2002; Schnittker 2017; Whooley 2019.

25. Currently, psychoanalytic psychiatrists lack formal representation within the APA after a series of reorganizations resulted in the elimination, in 2009, of the Committee on Psychotherapy by Psychiatrists (Mintz 2019).

26. For the history and tenets of interpersonal psychotherapy, see Klerman et al. 1984; Markowitz and Weissman 2012; Weissman, Markowitz, and Klerman 2000. The success of CBT in transforming psychotherapy is indisputable—measured, for example, by the hundreds of clinical trials conducted to test its efficacy (e.g., A. Beck 2005; J. Beck 2011; Butler et al. 2006), by its success in clinical psychology (Pilgrim 2011), and by its adoption as the primary line of intervention prescribed by the NHS, Britain's national health system (Pickersgill 2019).

27. See, e.g., Hale 1995; Luhrmann 2000; Whooley 2019.

28. Psychiatry's turn to biology had many prominent advocates, including psychiatrist, neuroscientist, and Nobel Prize winner Eric Kandel (1998) who published a (conciliatory) call for greater investment in this arena in the pages of the *American Journal of Psychiatry*. For an ethnographic account of the transition from psychodynamic to biological psychiatry in the late 1980s and early 1990s, see Luhrmann 2000.

29. We understand and try to treat our "everyday suffering" biologically, argues Davis (2020), and the psychiatric profession along with pharmaceutical companies have gained from turning "distress" in the face of life events into "disorder," to borrow sociologist Allan Horwitz's (2007) formulation. Statistic from Terlizzi and Norris 2021.

30. This was at about 10 percent in 2020, according to the same survey results (Terlizzi and Norris 2021).

31. Just as the DSM-5, the manual's latest revision, was appearing in press, Thomas Insel, then director of NIMH, declared that the NIMH would be moving "away from DSM categories" (quoted in Whooley 2019, 191) and adopting a new system of classification called the Research Domain Criteria (for a sociological analysis of these and other controversies surrounding the DSM-5, see Whooley 2014, 2016). Additionally, new research has raised questions about the effectiveness of antidepressant medications, some of the most widely prescribed group of drugs in the field. See, e.g., Goldberg et al. 2019; Kirsch 2010; Maslej et al. 2020; Sanacora 2020.

32. Mellman and Beresin 2003.

33. Mellman and Beresin 2003.

34. Miller, Scully, and Winstead 2003, 129.

35. Mellman and Beresin 2003, 149.

36. Miller, Scully, and Winstead 2003, 129. Though board certification is not required to practice medicine in the US—a medical license obtained after medical school is the necessary credentialing standard—it is typically required by employers or insurance agencies (ABPN 2018). As of 2017, psychiatrists are assessed during residency on clinical skills that include: the physician-patient relationship, the psychiatric interview, and the case presentation (ABPN 2017).

37. Mohl, Lomax, Tasman, Chan, Sledge, et al. 1990, 11. Paul Mohl and his co-authors were not simply expressing their personal views. They were representing the findings of a joint working group of the Association for Academic Psychiatry and the American Association of Directors of Psychotherapy Training.

38. Mohl, Lomax, Tasman, Chan, Sledge, et al. 1990, 11–12.

39. Mohl, Lomax, Tasman, Chan, Sledge, et al. 1990, 7. Debates about the relevance of psychotherapy to psychiatric training and practice continue. Belcher (2020) offers a view of that imagined "future psychiatrist" from the present; Morisette and Fleisher (2021) argue for the continued import of psychotherapy to psychiatric practice.

40. Miller, Scully, and Winstead 2003, 128; see also Beresin and Mellman 2002; Berlim and Turecki 2007; Swing 2007. The structure of residency education is partly a function of requirements by the ACGME and partly dependent on the resources of training programs. Established in 1981 as an independent nonprofit organization, the ACGME is central to physicians' self-governance and legitimacy. The organization regulates physician education during residency and fellowship across specialties by setting and enforcing standards. In psychiatry, as in other medical subfields, such standards are decided upon by a Residency Review Committee (the Psychiatry RRC) and have long included hospital and clinic-based training in pharmacological and therapeutic interventions. Yet this relative stability belies a history of contentious debates about psychiatric training that reflect tensions in psychiatry's identity as a profession and its relationship to the broader domain of medicine.

41. "Competence" and its assessment have long vexed medical educators (for some discussions in psychiatry, see, e.g., Giordano and Briones 2003; Khurshid et al. 2005; Swick, Hall, and Beresin 2006). Sociologist Mary-Jo DelVecchio Good ([1995] 1998) has written the defining social scientific analysis on the topic. For further discussion, see chapter 7.

42. Yager, Kay, and Mellman 2003, 126, see also Mohl 2004.

43. Yager, Kay, and Mellman 2003, 126.

44. Conflicts were especially pronounced around the turn of the twenty-first century, a time when the field of medicine as a whole and psychiatry alongside it were in the throes of a transition to an evidentiary regime based on RCTs. The relative dearth of RCTs documenting psychodynamic therapy's successes in the early years of the twenty-first century was especially problematic. In contrast, CBT, DBT, and IPT were all viewed as "evidence-based."

45. Exchange cited in Boat et al. 2003, 63–64.

46. ACGME 2013, 13.

47. ACGME 2013, 13.

48. ACGME 2020, 2023; Guerrero et al. 2020.

49. ACGME 2023, 20.

50. ACGME 2020, 10.

51. ACGME 2020, 10.

52. AGME 2020, 4.

53. A recent example involves changes in the number of hours residents can work over a week and how this change has been implemented; see, e.g., Kellogg 2011; Szymczak and Bosk 2012. The shift to "evidence-based" practice has also raised questions about how new standards get implemented: see Greenhalgh et al. 2008; McGlynn et al. 2003; Timmermans and Angell 2001; Timmermans and Berg 2003.

For other discussions of how professionals respond to changes in work standards, see, e.g., DiBenigno 2018; Kellogg 2014; Lampland and Star 2009.

54. Luhrmann 2000, 25.

55. The residents master DSM categories with relative ease. In Luhrmann's study, novice psychiatrists prided themselves on the speed with which they could arrive at a diagnosis after observing a patient for mere seconds (2000, 34–41). Moreover, whereas psychiatry residents begin learning about psychotropic medications in medical school, during residency they become specialists in some types of conditions and classes of medications.

56. Luhrmann 2000, 50. Other scholars have complicated this view. Jonathan Metzl (2003) aptly pointed out that the "new doctorhood" of biological psychiatry that emerged with the advent of psychotropic medications depended less on "the talking skills of psychotherapy" and more on the "writing skills involved in prescription" (26). This reconfiguration of psychiatric practice represented a fundamentally different form of expertise. In biopsychiatry, Metzl argues, knowledge and authority are split between the prescriber and their tools. As psychiatrists shifted from talking to prescribing, Metzl proposed, their expertise receded from view, allowing the drugs themselves to become the principal agents in patients' betterment. Nevertheless, as the residents see their patients coming to the hospital deeply troubled and leaving it in a calmer and more contained state, they view themselves as doing what doctors do: relieving pain.

57. For a description of psychoanalysis and its principles, see Freud 1961, 1963; for an overview of psychoanalytic schools, Mitchell and Black 1995; for the history of psychoanalysis in American psychiatry, see, e.g., Hale 1971, 1995; Schechter 2014; Whooley 2019.

58. Gabbard 2004, 3.

59. Nancy Chodorow, a psychoanalyst and trained sociologist, offers an illuminating discussion of transference (1999, esp. ch. 1). For some psychoanalytic writing on the topic, see Freud 1961, esp. 56–58; Gabbard 2004; Goldstein 2000; Jacobs 1991, 1999; Ogden 1992; Orr 1954.

60. Gabbard 2004, 3.

61. A. Beck 1963, 1964. Though the history of cognitive behavior therapy is frequently traced to the work of psychiatrist Aaron Beck (see, e.g., Weishaar 1993), its beginnings are more muddled. Cognitive therapy emerged simultaneously in the work of Beck and psychologist Albert Ellis, who named his approach rational-emotive therapy (Arnkoff and Glass 1992); Beck even references Ellis's work as an influence. Both Beck and Ellis drew on their psychoanalytic training as they developed their interventions, and both emphasized the importance of *conscious* thoughts in the experience and treatment of mental illness. Finally, both stressed the need to change patients' irrational beliefs (see, e.g., Rosner 2012, 2014, 2018; Stark 2017). Despite sharing credit for this new approach, Beck cut a more compelling figure to represent the movement: his emphasis on empirical evidence and scientific testing fit with the turn in the 1970s and '80s toward these values in medicine broadly and psychiatry in particular.

62. Beck 1964, 571.

63. Beck 1964, 568. The process is, Beck made clear early on, driven by a commitment to objectivity and rationality: "The procedure consists essentially of the application of the rules of evidence and logic to the cognitions and the consideration of alternative explanations or interpretations by the patient" (1964, 569).

64. See Arnkoff and Glass 1992; Glass and Arnkoff 1992.

65. Knorr Cetina 1999.

66. P. Haas 1992.

67. Following Renee Fox (1957, 1980), researchers typically subsumed such conundrums under the umbrella of uncertainty. Medical trainees, Fox argued, have to manage their knowledge of their own limitations, as well as the inherent boundaries of medical knowledge along with the ever-expanding amount of medical facts. The residents I spent time with undoubtedly experienced uncertainty as they learned to doctor with or without drugs. But focusing on uncertainty alone elides the peculiarities of their positions upon entering psychotherapy training: they did so as already trained biopsychiatrists. They were not simply novices, ready to complete the main rites of passage of the program. Nor can the skepticism and ambivalence they brought to psychotherapy be reduced to what sociologist Donald Light (1979, 1980) has described as techniques for controlling uncertainty or what Jack Haas and William Shaffir (1977, 1982) have characterized as adopting a cloak of competence. More than the management of uncertainty, their training was defined by the management of doubt born out of the epistemic and professional frictions embedded in their roles.

68. The literature on professional socialization is extensive. Examples include Anteby 2013; Becker et al. 1961; Bosk 1979; Coser 1979; DelVecchio Good (1995) 1998; Gill 2009; Good 1994; Jenkins 2020; Light 1980; Luhrmann 2000; Merton, Reader, and Kendall 1957; Mertz 2007; Prentice 2013; Van Maanen 1973, 1975. For a systemic overview, see Anteby, Chan, and DiBenigno 2016; Gorman and Sandefur 2011. A vast majority of earlier studies of professionalization (including those of postgraduate education) were conducted in settings where there was little disagreement about the profession's object of knowledge and the best ways, to use sociologist Andrew Abbott's (1988) definition of *expert work*, to diagnose it, treat it, and think about it. Even as innovation may challenge such agreement (e.g., Menchik 2020; Owen-Smith 2001), professionals have agreed-upon means to adjudicate such challenges. Yet in the field of mental health, where professionals have distinct understandings of what mental illness is and how it should be treated, the opposite holds. See Jenkins 2020 for a discussion about the assumption of coherence of medicine; see also Anteby, Chan, and DiBenigno 2016 for other fields.

69. In medicine, "premed" undergraduates progress to medical school upon passing the Medical College Admission Test (MCAT); medical students can begin their clinical internships after successfully completing the United States Medical Licensing Examination (USMLE) Step 1, focused on the science of medicine, and then transition to yearlong internships after passing the USMLE Step 2, focused on clinical knowledge. Next, after passing the USMLE Step 3, which focuses on assessing skills necessary for working independently, interns formally begin residency—that is, their training in a medical specialty. Finally, after completing the residency, they can become "board-certified" physicians by passing the licensing exams in their field. See Jenkins 2020 for a discussion of this process.

70. Fox 1957, 1980.

71. Pratt, Rockman, and Kaufmann 2006.

72. Abbott 1988, 2.

73. For a review of the extensive literature on these topics, see Gorman and Sandefur 2011. Some examples include: Abbott 1988; Anteby 2008; Barley 1996; Bechky 2003a, 2003b; DiBenigno 2018; Dobbin and Kelly 2007; Kellogg 2011, 2014; Kellogg, Orlikowski, and Yates 2006; Timmermans 2005; Van Maanen and Barley 1984.

74. Whooley 2019.

75. For a similar perspective, see Anspach 1993; Luhrmann 2000.

76. Merton and Barber (1963) 1976, 6.

77. See, e.g., Frickel et al. 2016 on interdisciplinarity, Glaeser 2010 on political epistemics, and Waters 1990, 1994, 1999; Waters and Jiménez 2005 on immigrants' conundrums.

78. Merton and Barber (1963) 1976, 66.

79. Pratt, Rockman, and Kaufman 2006. For empirical illustrations of this phenomenon, see, e.g., DiBenigno 2018; Kellogg 2011, 2014.

80. Scholars of interdisciplinarity have shown that even in contexts defined by a commitment to superseding boundaries, they nevertheless remain in place (Downey et al. 2016; Frickel, Albert, and Prainsack 2016; Smith-Doerr et al. 2019). Friction is a defining characteristic of such work, as "strained interactions" (Downey et al. 2016) between participants in interdisciplinary teams must be worked through. Professional identity and disciplinary training shape practical engagements even in the most committed groups. For other settings in which professionals must adapt to new work demands, see Anteby 2008; Anteby and Holm 2021; Baumgart-McFarland, Chiarello, and Slay 2022; Kellogg 2011, 2014.

81. Skepticism is rarely explicitly discussed or sociologically analyzed in such works. It is most frequently subsumed under distrust (e.g., Hardin 2002), or doubt and disbelief (e.g., Smilde 2007). In the realm of politics, it is described as a source of division that needs to be overcome (e.g., Bennett et al. 2013).

82. Merton (1973) proposed that science is governed by four norms: communism, universalism, disinterestedness, and organized skepticism. For a contemporary elaboration of "civil skepticism," see Ramírez-i-Ollé 2018. For a reconsideration of Mertonian norms, see Panofsky 2010.

83. Stengers 1997, 158.

84. Not all residents engaged in practical displays of doubt in the group meetings, nor did they all do so to the same extent. Nevertheless, expressions of doubt were frequent enough and drew enough agreement from the groups I observed that I came to view skepticism as an essential dimension of the residents' roles. For a parallel discussion of the personal traits that make some people more likely to believe in what T. M. Luhrmann calls "invisible others" in a religious context, see Luhrmann 2020, esp. 58–78.

85. In "Fixation of Belief," Peirce (1991) argued that scientific inquiry is the best path from doubt to "belief." I highlight instead the socioinstitutional conditions that not only make skepticism likely but also facilitate its resolution. I thank Owen Whooley for bringing Peirce's writing on this topic to my attention.

86. Goffman 1959, 13.

87. For a compelling discussion of the analytical productivity of such meetings for organizational researchers, see Kunda 1992; Owen-Smith 2001.

Chapter Two

1. Davydow and his collaborators (2008) offer a similar report on another residency program. Zisook and colleagues (2011) track psychiatry residents' interest in psychotherapy across several residencies.

2. The Community Mental Health Centers Act was one of the key pieces of legislation leading to deinstitutionalization (Grob 1994).

3. For an in-depth description of the profession at the time, see Hale 1995.

4. For a discussion of the financial pressures that have shaped mental health care, see Grob 1994; Mechanic 1998, 2008; Stevens 1989.

5. Details about this federal initiative can be viewed online; see Library of Congress 2022.

6. The guidelines have become more prescriptive over time. The current standards (ACGME 2023, 28) state: "Each resident must have significant experience treating outpatients longitudinally for at least one year, to include initial evaluation and treatment of ongoing individual psychotherapy patients, some of whom should be seen weekly."

7. See, e.g., Gabbard 2007; Gabbard and Kay 2001; Kay 1996; Kay and Myers 2014; Mellman 2006; Mellman and Beresin 2003; Miller, Scully, and Winstead 2003; Mohl, Lomax, Tasman, Chan, Sledge, et al. 1990; Reiser 1988; Yager and Bienenfeld 2003; Yager, Kay, and Mellman 2003; Yager et al. 2005.

8. For recent discussion of this shift, see Underman and Hirshfield 2016; Vinson and Underman 2020.

9. The transition from medical school to residency centers on what is commonly known as "the match"(National Resident Matching Program 2023). For a discussion of the sociological dimensions of this process, see Jenkins 2020.

10. The internship year (PGY-1) includes a range of clinical rotations, not all focused on the particular specialization the medical graduate will undertake during PGY-2 (see, e.g., description from Husarewycz, Fleisher, and Skakum 2015 for psychiatry).

11. Luhrmann 2000, 90.

12. The major change the DSM-5 (American Psychiatric Association 2013) introduced to diagnosing mental disorder was the elimination of the multiaxial system codified in previous versions of the manual. No longer differentiated into clinical disorders (Axis I), personality disorders (Axis II), and other medical conditions (Axis III), mental health diagnoses are listed together, in order of "clinical importance." Psychosocial factors (Axis IV) are listed with the diagnoses, while the Global Assessment of Functioning (GAF) scale (Axis V) has been replaced by the WHO Disability Assessment Schedule (WHODAS).

13. A text revision of the DSM-IV (the DSM-IV-TR) was published in 1994 and was in use at the time of my fieldwork. The DSM enumeration switched from Roman to Arabic numbers beginning with the DSM-5.

14. Whether patients themselves view their hospital stays as "being taken care of" is another matter. For critical accounts see, e.g., Estroff 1981; Goffman 1961. For a more positive, contemporary firsthand account, see Antrim 2021.

15. Psychiatrists come to see the DSM as a flexible guide and, as sociologist Owen Whooley (2010) found in his study of more experienced practitioners, deploy its diagnostic categories nimbly, aware of insurance requirements and the stigma associated with certain diagnoses.

16. Information retrieved from the NIMH (2022).

17. The challenges of such "split" roles have received some attention in the psychiatric literature—for example, Goin 2001; J. Mark 2001.

18. Unlike the process of identifying patients whom they could treat pharmacologically, finding patients for psychotherapy was less straightforward, requiring the help of instructors and more experienced residents. Typically, this involved identifying

patients who, in addition to taking psychiatric medications, could also be good candidates for psychotherapy. For example, a patient coming to the clinic suffering from depression could be a good patient for psychodynamic psychotherapy in addition to being prescribed an SSRI. Another who sought help for anxiety may receive a prescription and a recommendation that they start CBT treatment.

19. See Mullen et al. 2004. The milestone framework replaced this method of assessing the residents' psychodynamic knowledge.

20. In their classic study of medical school, Becker and his coauthors (1961) reveal students' intense preoccupation with time and their schedules. Closer to the contemporary moment, scholars have shown that this preoccupation endures after this early training stage, shaping the residency as well as, more significantly, how doctors conceive of what it means to be not only a dedicated student but also a good doctor (e.g., Kellogg 2011; Szymack and Bosk 2012).

21. When I spoke to Leah during her third year, she described a schedule split among "clinics"—namely, meetings focused on particular diagnoses (such as anxiety disorders or bipolar disorder) or psychiatric populations (such as child psychiatry, geriatric psychiatry, or perinatal patients)—didactic rotations (including "grand rounds" and the psychotherapy meetings), and "return visits" dedicated to medication management.

22. For research on changes in residents' temporal commitments, see Kellogg 2011, 2014; Szymczak and Bosk 2012.

23. In this respect, Shorewood stood out from other programs in how it implemented the ACGME requirements for psychotherapy training. In a recent study, Rim, Cabaniss, and Topor (2020) found that a majority of psychiatry residencies (in a sample of 79, a little less than half of all residencies at the time) do not have dedicated "psychotherapy tracks" for their residents and do not offer them didactic instruction and supervision in the care of patients.

24. Notable examples of social scientific writing on time and temporality include Auyero 2011; Dubinskas 1988; Fine 1990; Flaherty 2002; Roth 1963; Schwartz 1974; Zerubavel 1979, 1982.

Chapter Three

1. This conundrum has some parallels with the distinction social scientists draw between "illness" and "disease." To borrow from Kleinman (1988, 7), *illness* "refers to the patient's perception, experience, expression, and pattern of coping with symptoms," while *disease* is "the way [medical] practitioners recast illness in terms of their theoretical models of pathology."

2. The DSM-5 defines OCD as a condition in which individuals have obsessions, compulsions, or both, that they try to contain or repress.

3. Social scientists have written extensively about the dilemmas professionals must navigate when putting abstract knowledge into practice (e.g., Clarke and Fujimura 1992; Fujimura 1987; Goodwin 1994; Seron and Silbey 2009). In medicine this means making sense of each patient's illness in the diagnostic and treatment terms of the profession (e.g., Abbott 1988; Freidson 1970; Whooley 2010). Thus, the dictum that "every patient is different" can hold just as easily in pharmacology, where the residents have to make sense of patients' idiosyncrasies in terms that link biology, behavior, and pharmaceuticals. Much of the work of pharmacology revolves around crafting a prescription that will address patients' unique reactions to drugs as well as

their symptoms. But whereas pharmacology discussions focus on the concrete effects of medications, psychotherapy's broader mandate opens up entirely new avenues for miscommunication and doubt.

4. The concept of *epistemic authority* has been largely implicit in much discussion of professional power. Following Stivers and Timmermans (2020), I use the term to highlight doctors' scientifically legitimated power in matters of knowledge about disease, its course, and its resolution. Physicians exercise their epistemic authority through the acts of diagnosis, treatment, and prescribing, though, as Epstein (1996), Stivers and Timmermans (2020), and others have shown, patients do not simply accept their pronouncements without contestation. For related discussions of epistemic authority, see Starr 1982; Whooley 2013.

5. In an editorial published in the *Journal of Clinical Psychopharmacology*, Jose de Leon (2016) argued that pharmacogenetic tests are both "hyped" and misunderstood. In the same journal, a year earlier, Richard Shader (2015) criticized psychiatrists for embracing such tests so that they could "avoid" talking to patients. For social scientific perspectives on the search for biological causes of mental illness, see Harrington 2019; Navon 2019; Navon and Eyal 2016.

6. Doubts about patients' reports may be said to be the case in any profession that deals in what sociologist Everett Hughes (1958, 78–87) called "guilty knowledge": knowledge of their clients' sins, crimes, hatreds, sicknesses; in one word, secrets. Even as such professionals—the priest, the lawyer, the physician, the journalist, the scientist, the scholar, the diplomat, to name some of Hughes's examples—have a license to work with such knowledge, distrust is built into their relationships with clients and, Hughes argues, with society more broadly. This distrust is partly what accreditation rules, codes of ethics, and other governance tools are meant to address.

7. In a conversation analytic study, Bergmann (1992) showed that psychiatrists can use uncertainty to get patients to provide more information about their problems.

8. Porter (1995, 5), argued that our contemporary understanding of "objectivity" is the product of sociohistorical forces that have fueled a "trust in numbers." "Mechanical objectivity" in his framework refers to following epistemic rules about how and when to employ numbers; in contrast, "disciplinary objectivity" is tied to expert consensus and moral commitments.

9. I borrow the term *inscriptive* from science and technology scholarship (e.g., Latour and Woolgar 1979), where it refers to the results of the ubiquitous writing practices that scientists engage in to discipline nature, construct facts, and claim credibility. In medicine, these forms have become increasingly popular outside the realm of psychiatry proper: they are routinely employed, for example, in annual visits to primary care physicians and in insurance coverage determinations.

10. Winfield (2022) explains that the act of "interpellation"—compelling an actor to take on an identity (in this case, that of patient)—can take place both publicly and privately. In psychiatry, close and intimate conversations between doctors and patients can function as powerful—though not always successful—conduits for patients' disclosure. Standardized forms structure how patients describe and understand their experiences. They also delimit doctors' own attention, facilitating a particular kind of expert work.

11. There is an extensive literature documenting the effects of stigma on those suffering from mental illness, originating with Erving Goffman's (1963) seminal work, *Stigma: Notes on the Management of Spoiled Identity*. Recent research is summarized by Pescosolido and Martin (2015) and Link and Phelan (2017).

12. Carr and Obertino-Norwood (2022) have argued that "evidence-based practice" has become a "complex system of legitimation." In psychotherapy, CBT practitioners can point to hundreds of randomized clinical trials establishing the efficacy of their approaches (reviewed and summarized by Butler et al. 2006; David, Cristea, and Hofmann 2018; Hofmann, Asmundson, and Beck 2013; van Dis et al. 2020); psychodynamic research has also been catching up (see, e.g., Gabbard, Gunderson, and Fonagy 2002; Leichsenring 2005, 2009; Leichsenring and Rabung 2008, 2011; Leichsenring, Hiller, et al. 2006, 2013, Leichsenring, Leweke, et al. 2015; Leichsenring and Steinert 2017; Leuzinger-Bohleber and Kachele 2015; Shedler 2010). There is also a substantial literature that indicates no significant difference in outcomes between psychotherapeutic approaches (e.g., Cuijpers, van Straten, Schuurmans, and van Oppen 2008; Cuijpers, van Straten, Schuurmans, van Oppen, et al. 2010; Luborsky, Singer, and Luborsky 1975; M. Smith and Glass 1977; Steinert et al. 2017; Wampold 2015).

13. The residents were not expected to pursue their own psychotherapy, and few were open about doing so. This is a contrasting picture compared with how residents approached personal therapy at the height of psychoanalytic dominance in the field (see, e.g., Hale 1995; Light 1980). A more recent survey of psychiatry residents revealed that about a third of survey respondents pursued personal therapy and that being part of a training program that had ties to a psychoanalytic institute as well as being further along in training were significantly associated with doing so (Haak and Kaye 2009).

14. See, e.g., Becker et al. 1961; Bosk 1979; Dreyfus and Dreyfus 2005.

15. For an elaboration of tacit knowledge in expert work, see, e.g., Collins 1974, 2010; Dreyfus and Dreyfus 2005.

16. The residents faced structural forces that compelled them to rely on the DSM: they were required to enter medical diagnoses into patients' records, which in turn were necessary for administrative purposes, not the least of which was payments from insurers.

17. See, e.g., Luhrmann 2000; Whooley 2010.

18. Exemplary works include Bowker and Star 1999; Fourcade 2009; Lampland and Star 2009; Porter 1995. Porter makes clear that quantification and standardization are a means for experts to establish their authority vis-à-vis other social actors.

Chapter Four

1. Eisenberg 1983.

2. The social scientific literature on boundary work is extensive. Informative reviews were authored by Lamont (1992), Lamont and Molnar (2002), and Pachucki, Pendergrass, and Lamont (2007). In science studies, some of the foundational work on the topic is by Thomas Gieryn (1983, 1999).

3. See Carr 2010 for a review of apprenticeship in expertise acquisition. In psychoanalytic training, "candidates," as novices are called, must undergo their own psychoanalysis. This is useful partly because it gives them direct access to seeing an experienced analyst in action.

4. Coser (1961) was largely concerned with illuminating the connections between observability and social conformity. My focus here is instead on the conundrums of apprenticing in a craft that you cannot directly and repeatedly observe. For an elaboration of the relationships among visibility, autonomy, and conformity, see Bosk 1979 on surgery residency, Anspach 1988 on the case presentation as a mode

of supervision. Jenkins (2020) has also written persuasively about the importance of supervision and apprenticing for physicians.

5. Freidson 1970.

6. Though there was less reticence to conduct such activities in this orientation compared with psychodynamic training, direct observation was nevertheless not routinely practiced. The only exception were treatments that residents conducted in front of one-way mirrors in the rotation focused on CBT for children and adolescents. While instructive in their own right, such sessions did not serve the same instructional purpose nor had the same legitimating effects as those conducted by experienced clinicians themselves.

7. Burns's book *Feeling Good: The New Mood Therapy* was originally published in 1980 and was one of the first to introduce CBT to the general public. With more than four thousand reviews on the online seller Amazon and a nearly perfect five-star rating from enthusiastic consumers, the book promises "the clinically proven, drug-free treatment for depression." (Information about book rating retrieved December 1, 2020, from https://www.amazon.com/Feeling-Good-New-Mood-Therapy/dp/0380731762/ref=tmm_pap_swatch_0?_encoding=UTF8&qid=1607362631&sr=8-1.) A second edition was published in 1999. Burns also recently published *Feeling Great: The Revolutionary New Treatment for Depression and Anxiety* (2020).

8. I borrow the phrase "clinical empathy" from sociologists Vinson and Underman (2020), who contrast this newer standard of affective engagement in medical care to earlier standards around "detached concern." Underman and Hirshfield (2016) also offer a useful review of this shift.

9. Sociologist Andrew Abbott (1988) has argued that all expert work consists of diagnosis (defining a problem in the terms of a particular professional group), inference (thinking about it), and treatment (solving the problem with the tools of the group). While diagnosis and treatment can be observed, inference is the most challenging to track empirically, partly because it happens in cognitive or embodied ways that are not always visible to the researcher.

10. Harry M. Collins (1974, 2010) has elaborated the concept of "tacit knowledge," drawing inspiration from the work of Michael Polanyi ([1958] 1962), who called it "personal knowledge." Others have also described tacit knowledge as essential to claiming expertise (Collins and Evans 2007; Dreyfus and Dreyfus 2005) and have sought to shed light on its acquisition (e.g., Goodwin 1994; Rose-Greenland 2013).

11. The resident and I had different frames of reference. I compared Robert's session with the psychodynamic ones I had witnessed earlier in my fieldwork. For Aaron, the point of comparison was a fifteen-minute medication management appointment.

12. By "9/11," the patient, Terry, and the residents were referring to the September 11, 2001, terrorist attacks that took place in New York City; Washington, DC; and Philadelphia (for a description of the events, see Arkin 2021).

13. Albert Ellis is recognized as one of the founders of cognitive and behavioral approaches through his elaboration of rational emotive behavior therapy (REBT); see Stark 2017; Weinrach 1988. Doctors Judith Beck and her father, Aaron Beck, in 1994 cofounded the Beck Institute in Philadelphia, the top organization in the US for training in CBT, where Judith Beck currently serves as president; see Beck Institute n.d.

14. Whether they themselves prescribed medications in addition to doing therapy (as was the case for Terry, a psychiatrist and psychoanalyst) or worked with psychiatrists who managed the pharmaceutical side of treatment (as was the case for

the psychologists and social workers in the program), these clinicians, too, had experienced the epistemic mismatches between biopsychiatry and psychotherapy.

15. Lamont and Molnar 2002, 168. Social scientific writing on boundaries is extensive. Notable works include Bourdieu 1991; M. Douglas 1966; Durkheim (1912) 1995; Lamont 1992.

16. There is a considerable literature on boundary work in professions and science. Gieryn (1983, 1999) wrote some of the foundational work on what he called the "cultural boundaries of science." Other scholars have examined boundary work in various occupations (e.g., Anteby 2010; Bechky 2003; DiBenigno 2018; Halpern 1992; Mizrachi and Shuval 2005; Vallas 2001).

17. See, e.g., Abbass et al. 2014; Beutel et al. 2010.

18. This observation is not unique to Shorewood. Many specialists in psychiatry continue to question the value of psychoanalysis or psychodynamic training, and hospitals in which residents are trained function as principal battlegrounds. For a survey of residents' perceptions of this matter at various sites, see Calabrese et al. 2010. For a first-person account, see Klitzman 1995.

19. Sulloway 1992. For a more nuanced argument, see Guenther 2015.

20. For a discussion of psychoanalysis in France, see Roudinesco 1990, 2016; in Argentina, see Lakoff 2005b.

21. Psychotherapy is a crowded field. For an overview of some of the most significant approaches, see, e.g., Freedheim 1992, esp. part 1; Prochaska and Norcross 2013.

22. See, e.g., A. Beck 1976; Rosner 2012, 2014.

23. Of the more than two dozen psychoanalysts and psychodynamic psychotherapists I interviewed, only one described an ongoing treatment that had lasted more than ten years and seemed to approximate the "indefinite" time frame Robert disavowed. The rest described treatments that lasted closer to two or three years. Moreover, I had spoken with more than a dozen CBT practitioners during my research who told me of treatments that extended well past the initial two- to three-month time frame, or whose patients returned for regular "tune-ups."

24. See, e.g., Carr 2010; Goodwin 1994; Lave and Wenger 1991; Rose-Greenland 2013.

25. Shapin 1984. This credibility accounts for the power of visualizing technologies in establishing facts and their "objectivity" (Daston and Galison 1992, 2007). It also, as Shapin has argued (see Shapin 1984, 1995; Shapin and Schaffer 1985), explains the importance of particular "literary technologies" that seek to make laboratory findings "known to those who were not direct witnesses" (Shapin 1984, 484). For a feminist critique and elaboration of "witnessing," see Haraway 1988, 1997.

Chapter Five

1. According to the *Diagnostic and Statistical Manual of Mental Disorders: DSM-5-TR*, generalized anxiety disorder manifests itself in excessive worries and a difficulty to control them, and can be identified through symptoms of restlessness, fatigue, difficulty concentrating, irritability, muscle tension, and sleep disturbance (American Psychiatric Association 2022).

2. Selective serotonin reuptake inhibitors (SSRIs) are a class of psychotropics most commonly prescribed for the treatment of depression, anxiety, and other mood disorders. The US Food and Drug Administration offers an informative description of the class of drugs, including generics, name brands, and drug effects; see FDA 2014.

3. Carr 2021, 529.

4. The social scientific scholarship on medical socialization includes classics such as Anspach 1988; Becker et al. 1961; Bosk 1979; DelVecchio Good (1995) 1998; Good 1994; and more recent contributions by Jenkins (2020), Kellogg (2011), and Prentice (2013). For an informative discussion of the differences between professional identity and expertise, see Eyal 2013.

5. In attending to such meetings, I also build on work by organizational scholars who have argued for their analytical significance. Notable examples include Kunda 1992; Owen-Smith 2001.

6. His doubts were not unfounded. During my fieldwork and in interviews with nearly two dozen cognitive behavioral therapists, I learned that the main struggle they faced had to do with patients' ability and willingness to do "homework." This is also a major theme in the effectiveness literature concerning this approach. For a meta-analysis, see Kazantzis, Lampropoulos, and Deane 2005; Kazantzis et al. 2016.

7. Goffman 1959, 1961.

8. Nora had already provided all of us with handouts on DBT skills, and the residents (and I) were expected to remember these and put them into practice. Mindfulness skills include observing, describing, and *wise mind* (balancing emotions and rationality). The foundational work in this approach is by Marsha Linehan (Linehan 1993; Linehan, Ward-Ciesielski, and Neacsiu 2012), a clinician whose skills books are widely used (including at Shorewood).

9. A study published in 2009 found that, nationally, about a third of psychiatry residents pursue personal psychotherapy (Haak and Kaye 2009). Most frequently, such residents attended programs that had connections with a psychoanalytic institute; perhaps as a consequence, most were in psychodynamic psychotherapy.

10. Celexa is an SSRI prescribed largely to treat depression but also used at times for certain forms of anxiety. Zoloft is also an SSRI.

11. Damian found this especially problematic because the patient had come across Luvox, an SSRI approved by the FDA for the treatment of OCD but that had fallen out of favor among psychiatrists at the time.

12. Ativan, a brand name for the generic medication lorazepam, is part of a class of psychotropics known as benzodiazepines approved to treat anxiety and related disorders.

13. Ibarra 1999.

14. Carr 2021, 529.

Chapter Six

1. T. M. Luhrmann (2000), too, pointed out in her ethnography of psychiatric training in the 1980s and '90s the emphasis on clinical case discussions—these reflected, she argued, the residents' own preferences for knowledge that they could implement with their patients.

2. The arrangement was common, and the departing residents—more experienced and more cognizant of their patients' needs—spent time discussing such transitions with Terry and Patricia as well as with the junior residents who might take on their patients.

3. This estimate of "thirty times" is seemingly incongruous with a later description he gave about how long he had been treating Chloe—but in this larger number Jacob included the medication appointments they'd also had.

4. Psychoanalysts see patients' temporal infractions as attempts at avoiding the work of identifying what ails them; according to psychoanalytic thought, much of this avoidance happens unconsciously (e.g., Eissler 1974; Freud 1963; Furlong 1992).

5. For a discussion of how experts—psychotherapists in particular—use their emotions in their work, see Craciun 2018.

6. Freud (1961, 39) argued that "slips of the tongue" (along with difficulties in recalling names and losing things) "are not so insignificant as people, by a sort of conspiracy of silence, are ready to suppose." Rather, he continued, they "always have a meaning [. . . giving] expression to impulses and intentions which have to be held back and hidden from one's own consciousness." For this reason, he proposed, they ought to be investigated in the psychoanalytic encounter.

7. In invoking the notion of a "relational object," Lucas draws on a school of psychoanalysis identified as "object relations" championed by analysts such as W. R. D. Fairbarn, D. W. Winnicott, Michael Balint, and John Bowlby (discussed in Mitchell and Black 1995, 112–28).

8. Somers and Gibson (1994, 59, emphasis in original) argue that narratives are "*constellations of relationships* (connected parts), embedded in *time and space*, constituted by *causal emplotment*." This latter act—positioning episodes in relation to each other rather than broader categories—renders them significant. For the residents, narratives about their work with patients are akin to what Somers and Gibson (1994, 61) call "ontological narratives," stories they tell about who they are that are deeply connected with what they do.

9. Good 1994, esp. 65–87; see also Anspach 1988. For an overview of research and a conceptualization of "sensemaking," see Weick, Sutcliffe, and Obstfeld 2005.

10. Weick, Sutcliffe, and Obstfeld 2005, 409.

11. Anspach 1988, 357.

12. For a discussion of competence, see, for example, Becker et al. 1961; Bosk 1979; DelVecchio Good (1995) 1998.

13. Emirbayer 1997; Somers and Gibson 1994.

14. Glaeser 2011, 263.

Chapter Seven

1. The phrase originates in a video that Robert, the CBT for depression instructor, showed the residents in that rotation. In the video, Judith Beck explains that CBT requires therapists to balance directiveness with following the patient's lead, a challenge for novice and experienced therapists alike. In the same piece, Beck demonstrated how to implement this approach with a patient.

2. These considerations are not new: in 1915, Freud noted that what he called "transference-love" is "unavoidable" as well as "complicated" and "difficult to dissolve" (Freud 1963, 168). See also, e.g., Gabbard 1994; Saul 1962; Stefana 2017.

3. Gabbard 1994, 385.

4. The affinity between CBT and biopsychiatry has not gone unnoticed by pharmaceutical companies. About midway through the CBT for depression rotation, Turner (PGY-3) shared that "some of us got a book from Astra Zeneca about how to combine CBT and medications, and that was really helpful." The resident was aware of some of the potential implications of this outreach, explaining that "I don't know if this is good or not," in reference to receiving guidance from a corporation about how to treat patients. For a discussion of some of the moral conundrums medical students

navigate as they encounter the pharmaceutical industry, see Holloway 2014; Jibson 2006. Turner's admission further affirms the model of pragmatic accommodation that learning CBT makes possible for psychiatrists.

5. The brand-name medication Celexa is part of a group of psychotropics called selective serotonin reuptake inhibitors, SSRIs for short, commonly prescribed in the treatment of major depression.

6. Citalopram is the generic name for Celexa.

7. A resident proposed, jokingly, "He was thinking, time for CBT, or DBT, or PES!" Terry, the instructor, immediately offered, "For the physician or the patient?!" The jokes touched on the residents' fears of incompetence while also allowing them to vent their stress. Notable sociological writing on humor in professional training includes Coser 1979; Fox 1974.

8. DelVecchio Good (1995) 1998, 1.

9. For a discussion about how working with surrogate patients shapes medical students' understanding of their profession's "feeling" rules, see Underman 2020.

10. In addition to DelVecchio Good (1995) 1998, research on these topics includes Bosk 1979; Coser 1979; Good 1994; Kellogg 2011; Light 1980.

11. DelVecchio Good (1995) 1998, 124. DelVecchio Good ([1995] 1998, 200–201) notes that "when physicians try to specify exactly what these skills and knowledge are (what constitutes this medical expertise), this seemingly certain empirical domain appears enormously complex, nuanced, and far less precise." Indeed, in her prologue to the 1998 edition, she notes, "Science, research, knowledge, skills, trustworthiness, and responsibility to patients and health care teams are among the components of professional competence" (DelVecchio Good [1995] 1998, xiv).

12. In an ethnography of surgery residency, sociologist Charles Bosk (1979) showed that mistakes are implicitly assessed as either technical or normative, each with their own consequences for a resident's standing.

13. DelVecchio Good (1995) 1998, 131.

14. DelVecchio Good (1995) 1998, 148.

15. I borrow these terms from Ann Swidler's elaboration of the relationship between culture and action (Swidler 1986).

Chapter Eight

1. I borrow the phrase "social preconditions" from Mary Douglas (1984).

2. M. Douglas 1984, 80. Douglas (1984, 69) explicitly argues that, "to locate the sources of scepticism," one need not "survey [. . .] all the possible kinds of scepticism. It will not be necessary to distinguish the healthy scepticism of everyday life, nor the methodological doubt of epistemology, nor the scepticisms that do not threaten discourse, but rather make it possible." Instead, she argues that, rather than occupy themselves with creating a taxonomy of skepticisms, social scientists needs to focus on the conditions that make skepticism possible and lead to its entrenchment.

3. Elizabeth Lunbeck (1994) offers a detailed description of how psychiatrists worked with social workers in the Boston Psychopathic Hospital in the early decades of the twentieth century. For a discussion of the relationship between psychiatry and psychology, see, for example, how psychiatrists claimed psychoanalysis as their jurisdiction (Abbott 1988; Hale 1995) and the discussion of conflicts between psychiatrists and psychologists in Buchanan 2003. For a discussion of psychologists' current efforts at gaining prescription privileges, see American Psychological Association 2022.

4. This implicit commitment is made even more salient by psychiatrists' own sense of marginalization within the world of medicine, which, in turn, gives psychiatrists' claims to authority vis-à-vis psychologists and social workers renewed import.

5. However, as Mary Douglas (1984, 74) astutely observes, "sustained scepticism is a feasible stance for those who [. . .] stand apart from" society, a feat not easily achieved. Indeed, we must always understand skepticism and its champions and practitioners in the social contexts that foster or enable such a stance. Put differently, sustained skepticism is only possible in a community of like-minded peers that forgoes interaction with others around it.

6. Kellogg (2011) was concerned with the conditions that facilitated or, in turn, suppressed changes in medical education that imposed limits on residents' work hours.

7. In professional and scientific communities in particular, skepticism is constitutive of knowledge production and legitimation, as much of the science and technology scholarship has shown (for a useful introduction, see Shapin 1994). In one early formulation, Merton (1973) posited "organized skepticism" as an essential dimension of the ethos of science (see Ramírez-i-Ollé 2018 for an empirical elaboration).

8. M. Douglas 1984; Owen-Smith 2001.

9. For a compelling discussion of similar process in a scientific laboratory, see Owen-Smith 2001.

10. At Shorewood, this amounted to one or two residents per cohort (out of groups of eleven or twelve) who pursued further psychoanalytic training and tried to pursue professional careers in which they could continue to do psychotherapy.

11. See Tadmon and Olfson 2022.

12. In the 2010s, only a small percentage of psychiatrists (11 percent to 15 percent) exclusively dedicated their work to psychotherapy (Tadmon and Olfson 2022, 113), a rate that has not changed since about the 1980s. Tadmon and Olfson (2022) also found a pattern of stark segregation in the provision of psychotherapy by psychiatrists. Most who did provide psychotherapy were concentrated in the Northeast and worked almost exclusively with middle-class white patients. They also tended to practice in private offices with private pay. In contrast, psychiatrists practicing in nonmetropolitan areas in the South and Midwest, working with sicker and poorer patients, tended to work exclusively with psychopharmacological interventions.

13. A survey of Canadian psychiatrists practicing in British Columbia revealed that a majority still provide psychotherapy and are doing so at increasing rates (Hadjipavlou, Hernandez, and Ogrodniczuk 2015).

14. Tadmon and Olfson 2022, 113.

15. For practice guidelines, see American Psychiatric Association 2010; American Psychological Association 2019. Reviews of combining psychotropics and psychotherapy include Dougherty et al. 2018; Guidi and Fava 2021; Guidi, Tomba, and Fava 2016.

16. The psychiatric curriculum includes psychodynamic psychotherapy, cognitive behavioral therapy (CBT, of which dialectical behavioral therapy [DBT] is an offshoot), and supportive therapy. Unlike psychodynamic psychotherapy, CBT, or DBT, supportive therapy is centered largely on offering patients empathy and validation. Rather than formal instruction in the tenets of supportive therapy, Shorewood supervisors assumed that, in learning how to conduct a psychiatric interview and interact with patients, the residents would develop facility with the practices of supportive therapy. There was one exception to this; namely, in the seminar centered

on clinical skills that fell outside the bounds of my observations. Both psychodynamic and cognitive behavioral approaches required significant portions of the residents' time and prompted the kind of epistemic and professional frictions that stoked their skepticism. For a discussion of training in supportive therapy, see C. Douglas 2008; Lurie 1990; Moffic 1990; Mohl, Lomax, Tasman, Chan, and Summergrad 1990.

17. In a retrospective survey of psychiatry residents who graduated from a Canadian program where they began learning psychotherapy in the first year, Morrissette and colleagues (2020) found that whereas a vast majority of them (90.5 percent of respondents) found the training to be highly beneficial and an even larger percentage (95.2 percent) thought it should start in the first year; only 23.8 percent of respondents had a psychotherapy-oriented practice. In a survey of selected US psychiatry residencies, Kovach, Dubin, and Combs (2015) also concluded that residents wanted more psychotherapy training.

18. See also Luhrmann 2000.

19. In a survey of psychiatry residents in fifteen US-based programs, Lanouette and her collaborators (2011) found that these newly minted psychiatrists considered psychotherapy central to their professional identities, with a small majority planning to offer psychotherapy to their patients as part of their work.

20. Brown and colleagues (2019) offer a review of the concept of treatment resistance and its uses (see also Berlim and Turecki 2007; G. Parker et al. 2005; G. Parker and Graham 2015). Howes, Thase, and Pillinger (2022) estimate that treatment resistance affects 20 percent to 60 percent of all patients taking psychiatric medications.

21. Whooley (2019) offers a detailed analysis of psychiatry's long struggle with "ignorance" and its strategies of reinvention.

22. Abbott 1988, esp. ch. 10.

23. T. Mark, Levit, and Buck 2009.

24. These states include New Mexico (law passed in 2002), Louisiana (2004), Illinois (2014), Iowa (2016), Idaho (2017), and Colorado (2023), as reported by the American Psychological Association (2022).

25. Moran 2023. However, in one worrisome trend, psychiatry's popularity as a specialty has also correlated with a major decrease in its enrollment of international medical graduates (Chen et al. 2021; Virani et al. 2021). This, observers have warned, can have negative implications for the profession's ability to meet the needs of minority populations.

26. For a survey of contemporary psychiatrists' professional practices, see Tadmon and Olfson 2022. For a qualitative study of psychiatrists working in New York City and its environs, see D. Smith 2019.

27. The "biopsychosocial" model has long been a siren call for psychiatry. In the early 1900s, psychiatrist Adolf Meyer came to dominate the field with his commitment to eclecticism. Later, psychiatrist George Engel (1977) published a damning assessment in the pages of *Science*, arguing that biomedicine has led physicians, psychiatrists included, away from patients, focusing them solely and detrimentally on their diseases. The term has remained an important rallying point, particularly for those who argue against the pharmacological focus of contemporary psychiatry.

28. Kalin (2022, 78) was writing in the opening pages of a special issue in the *American Journal of Psychiatry* about multimodal approaches to mental illness. Ironically, the issue also included a piece by Tadmon and Olfson (2022) that showed contemporary psychiatrists' increasing focus on psychopharmacology.

29. Examples include Fink 1988; Gabbard 2007; Hartmann 1992; Mellman and Beresin 2003. For a discussion of the biopsychosocial approach in medicine see, Engel 1977; Silverman et al. 1983; Vasile et al. 1987.

30. Gabbard and Kay 2001, 1961.

31. Gabbard and Kay 2001, 1961.

32. In the United States, psychiatrists' professional organization is the American Psychiatric Association; for psychologists it is the American Psychological Association; the parallel one for social workers is the National Association of Social Workers.

33. Organizations dedicated to epistemic affinities include (but are not limited to) the American Psychoanalytic Association, the Association for Behavioral and Cognitive Therapies, the Clinical Social Work Association, the Society for Psychotherapy Research, the American Association for Marriage and Family Therapy, and Division 39 for psychoanalytic psychologists.

34. Eyal 2006.

35. For most, this meant setting up private practices or joining small group practices that allowed them to set aside hour-long windows of time to book psychotherapy patients, and that did not require them to bill insurance for their nonpharmacological services.

36. Galison (1999, 157) productively described such contexts as "trading zones," places where people from diverse epistemic subcultures engage in the practical activity of coordinating "action and belief."

37. I rely here on the distinction between empirical and theoretical "generalization" explained by Mario Small (2009).

38. A recent programmatic change in the field of medicine that posed challenges for the education of new physicians has been the transition to "evidence-based" practice in the early 1990s. Early on, physicians resisted the new model, condemning it for disregarding their hard-earned clinical experience. In the terms I have used in this book, the transition presented physicians with a shift in epistemic culture, one that posed its own challenges for training medical students and residents and resulted in new contradictions. Physicians turned, inevitably, to skepticism. For discussions of these conundrums, see Timmermans and Angell 2001; Timmermans and Berg 2003. For how a group of doctors dealt with changing work tasks as a result of the Affordable Care Act, see Kellogg 2014.

39. Frickel, Albert, and Prainsack 2017.

40. For recent examples, see, for example, Anteby 2010, on jurisdictional disputes between professional anatomists and independent organizations engaged in the sale of cadavers; Bechky 2020, on forensic scientists who must work with police and attorneys to bring DNA evidence to light while still maintaining their scientific standards; Timmermans 2006, on medical examiners who navigate pressures from families and public officials when making suicide determinations; DiBenigno and Kellogg 2014, on collaboration in US hospitals; DiBenigno 2018, 2020, on how mental health professionals are able to conduct their work in military environments.

41. For an influential treatise on jurisdictions, see Abbott 1988.

42. Eyal 2013.

43. Jason Owen-Smith conducted one of the few ethnographies investigating the workings of skepticism in expert work and showed that skepticism was "a solution to the problems of control, coordination, and evaluation raised by uncertain scientific work" (Owen-Smith 2001, 427). John Parker and Edward Hackett (2012) and

Meritxell Ramírez-i-Ollé (2018) focus on skepticism's expression and management in two scientific communities: resilience studies in ecology and dendroclimatology, respectively. Karen Locke, Karen Golden-Biddle, and Martha Feldman (2008) along with Gary Alan Fine (2019) have elaborated on the role of doubt in generating new research insights.

44. Anteby, Chan, and DiBenigno 2016.

45. Ibarra and Obodaru (2016) draw on work by Arnold van Gennep (1960) and Victor Turner (1969), the two anthropologists best known for their work on liminality and rituals of transition, to elaborate their concept.

REFERENCES

Abbass, Allan A., Sarah J. Nowoweiski, Denise Bernier, Robert Tarzwell, and Manfred E. Beutel. 2014. "Review of Psychodynamic Psychotherapy Neuroimaging Studies." *Psychotherapy and Psychosomatics* 83:142–47.

Abbott, Andrew. 1988. *The System of Professions: An Essay on the Division of Expert Labor*. Chicago: University of Chicago Press.

Accreditation Council for Graduate Medical Education (ACGME). 2013. *Program Requirements for Graduate Medical Education in Psychiatry*. Last modified June 9, 2013. https://www.acgme.org/globalassets/PDFs/400_psychiatry_RC.pdf.

———. 2020. *Psychiatry Milestones*. Last modified March 2020. https://www.acgme .org/globalassets/pdfs/milestones/psychiatrymilestones.pdf.

———. 2023. *Program Requirements for Graduate Medical Education in Psychiatry*. Updated July 1, 2023. https://www.acgme.org/globalassets/pfassets/programrequirements/400_psychiatry_2023.pdf.

American Board of Psychiatry and Neurology (ABPN). 2017. *Requirements for Clinical Skills Evaluation in Psychiatry*. Published November 2017. https://www.abpn.com/wp-content/uploads/2015/01/CSE-Psychiatry-2017.pdf.

———. 2018. *Frequently Asked Questions from the Public*. Published October 2018. https://www.abpn.com/wp-content/uploads/2015/07/General-Public-FAQ1.pdf.

American Psychiatric Association. 2010. "Practice Guideline for the Treatment of Patients with Major Depressive Disorder." Washington, DC: American Psychiatric Association.

———. 2013. *Diagnostic and Statistical Manual of Mental Disorders: DSM-5*. Washington, DC: American Psychiatric Association.

———. 2022. *Diagnostic and Statistical Manual of Mental Disorders: DSM-5-TR*. Washington, DC: American Psychiatric Association.

American Psychological Association. 2019. *APA Clinical Practice Guideline for the Treatment of Depression across Three Age Cohorts*. Published February 2019. https://www.apa.org/depression-guideline/guideline.pdf.

———. 2022. "About Prescribing Psychologists." Last updated January 2022. https://www.apaservices.org/practice/advocacy/authority/prescribing-psychologists.

Anspach, Renee R. 1988. "Notes on the Sociology of Medical Discourse: The Language of Case Presentation." *Journal of Health and Social Behavior* 29 (4): 357–75.

———. 1993. *Deciding Who Lives: Fateful Choices in the Intensive-Care Nursery*. Berkeley: University of California Press.

Anteby, Michel. 2008. *Moral Gray Zones: Side Productions, Identity, and Regulation in an Aeronautic Plant*. Princeton, NJ: Princeton University Press.

———. 2010. "Markets, Morals, and Practices of Trade: Jurisdictional Disputes in the U.S. Commerce in Cadavers." *Administrative Science Quarterly* 55 (4): 606–38.

———. 2013. *Manufacturing Morals: The Values of Silence in Business School Education.* Chicago: University of Chicago Press.

Anteby, Michel, Curtis Chan, and Julia DiBenigno. 2016. "Three Lenses on Occupations and Professions in Organizations: Becoming, Doing, and Relating." *Academy of Management Annals* 10 (1): 183–244.

Anteby, Michel, and Audrey L. Holm. 2021. "Translating Expertise across Work Contexts: U.S. Puppeteers Move from Stage to Screen." *American Sociological Review* 86 (2): 310–40.

Antrim, Donald. 2021. "Finding a Way Back from Suicide." *New Yorker,* August 16, 2021. https://www.newyorker.com/magazine/2021/08/16/finding-a -way-back-from-suicide.

Arkin, William M. 2021. *On That Day: The Definitive Timeline of 9/11.* New York: Public Affairs.

Arnkoff, Diane B., and Carol R. Glass. 1992. "Cognitive Therapy and Psychotherapy Integration." In Freedheim, *History of Psychotherapy,* 657–94.

Auyero, Javier. 2011. "Patients of the State: An Ethnographic Account of Poor People's Waiting." *Latin American Research Review* 46 (1): 5–29.

Barley, Stephen R. 1996. "Technicians in the Workplace: Ethnographic Evidence for Bringing Work into Organizational Studies." *Administrative Science Quarterly* 41 (3): 401–4.

Baumgart-McFarland, Madison, Elizabeth Chiarello, and Tayla Slay. 2022. "Reluctant Saviors: Professional Ambivalence, Cultural Imaginaries, and Deservingness Construction in Naloxone Provision." *Social Science & Medicine* 309 (2022): article no. 115230. https://doi.org/10.1016/j.socscimed.2022.115230.

Bechky, Beth. 2003a. "Object Lessons: Workplace Artifacts as Representations of Occupational Jurisdiction." *American Journal of Sociology* 109 (3): 720–52.

———. 2003b. "Sharing Meaning across Occupational Communities: The Transformation of Understanding on a Production Floor. " *Organization Science* 14 (3): 312–30.

———. 2020. *Blood, Powder, and Residue: How Crime Labs Translate Evidence into Proof.* Princeton, NJ: Princeton University Press.

Beck, Aaron T. 1963. "Thinking and Depression I: Idiosyncratic Content and Cognitive Distortions." *Archives of General Psychiatry* 9 (4): 324–33.

———. 1964. "Thinking and Depression II: Theory and Therapy." *Archives of General Psychiatry* 10 (6): 561–71.

———. 1976. *Cognitive Therapy and the Emotional Disorders.* New York: International Universities Press.

———. 2005. "The Current State of Cognitive Therapy: A 40-Year Retrospective." *Archives of General Psychiatry* 62 (9): 953–59.

Beck Institute. n.d. "History of Beck Institute." Accessed July 24, 2023. https:// beckinstitute.org/about/history-of-beck-institute/.

Beck, Judith S. 2011. *Cognitive Behavior Therapy: Basics and Beyond.* New York: Guilford Press.

Becker, Howard Saul, Blanche Geer, Everett C. Hughes, and Anselm L. Strauss. 1961. *Boys in White: Student Culture in Medical School.* Chicago: University of Chicago Press.

Belcher, Ren. 2020. "Psychotherapy and the Professional Identity of Psychiatry in the Age of Neuroscience. " *Academic Psychiatry* 44 (2): 227–30.

Bennett, Elizabeth A., Alissa Cordner, Peter Taylor Klein, Stephanie Savell, and Gianpaolo Baiocchi. 2013. "Disavowing Politics: Civic Engagement in an Era of Political Skepticism." *American Journal of Sociology* 119 (2): 518–48.

Beresin, Eugene, and Lisa Mellman. 2002. "Competencies in Psychiatry: The New Outcomes-Based Approach to Medical Training and Education." *Harvard Review of Psychiatry* 10 (3): 185–91.

Bergmann, Jorg R. 1992. "Veiled Morality: Notes on Discretion in Psychiatry." In *Talk at Work: Interaction in Institutional Settings*, edited by Paul Drew and John Heritage, 137–62. New York: Cambridge University Press.

Berlim, Marcelo T., and Gustavo Turecki. 2007. "What Is the Meaning of Treatment Resistant/Refractory Major Depression (TRD)? A Systematic Review of Current Randomized Trials." *European Neuropsychopharmacology* 17 (11): 696–707.

Beutel, Manfred E., Rudolf Stark, Hong Pan, David Silbersweig, and Sylvia Dietrich. 2010. "Changes of Brain Activation Pre-Post Short-Term Psychodynamic Inpatient Psychotherapy: An FMRI Study of Panic Disorder Patients." *Psychiatry Research* 184 (2): 96–104.

Boat, Thomas F., Kathleen M. Patchan, Michael T. Abrams, Institute of Medicine Board on Neuroscience and Behavioral Health, and Committee on Incorporating Research into Psychiatry Residency Training. 2003. *Research Training in Psychiatry Residency: Strategies for Reform.* Washington, DC: National Academies Press.

Bosk, Charles L. 1979. *Forgive and Remember: Managing Medical Failure.* Chicago: University of Chicago Press.

Bourdieu, Pierre. 1991. *Language and Symbolic Power.* Cambridge, MA: Harvard University Press.

Bowker, Geoffrey, and Susan Leigh Star. 1999. *Sorting Things Out: Classification and Its Consequences.* Cambridge, MA: MIT Press.

Brown, Sage, Katherine Rittenbach, Sarah Cheung, Gail McKean, Frank P. MacMaster, and Fiona Clement. 2019. "Current and Common Definitions of Treatment-Resistant Depression: Findings from a Systematic Review and Qualitative Interviews." *Canadian Journal of Psychiatry* 64 (6): 380–87.

Buchanan, Roderick D. 2003. "Legislative Warriors: American Psychiatrists, Psychologists, and Competing Claims over Psychotherapy in the 1950s." *Journal of the History of the Behavioral Sciences* 39 (3): 225–49.

Burns, David D. (1980) 1999. *Feeling Good: The New Mood Therapy.* New York: Avon Books.

———. 2020. *Feeling Great: The Revolutionary New Treatment for Depression and Anxiety.* Eau Claire, WI: PESI Publishing and Media.

Butler, Andrew C., Jason E. Chapman, Evan M. Forman, and Aaron T. Beck. 2006. "The Empirical Status of Cognitive-Behavioral Therapy: A Review of Meta-Analyses." *Clinical Psychology Review* 26 (1): 17–31.

Calabrese, Christina, Andres Sciolla, Sidney Zisook, Robin Bitner, Jeffrey Tuttle, and Laura B. Dunn. 2010. "Psychiatric Residents' Views of Quality of Psychotherapy Training and Psychotherapy Competencies: A Multisite Survey." *Academic Psychiatry* 34 (1): 13–20.

Carr, E. Summerson. 2010. "Enactments of Expertise." *Annual Review of Anthropology* 39 (1): 17–32.

———. 2021. "Learning How Not to Know: Pragmatism, (In)expertise, and the Training of American Helping Professionals." *American Anthropologist* 123 (3): 526–38.

Carr, E. Summerson, and Hannah Obertino-Norwood. 2022. "Legitimizing Evidence: The Trans-Institutional Life of Evidence-Based Practice." *Social Science & Medicine* 310 (October 2022): 115130. https://doi.org/10.1016/j.socscimed.2022.115130.

Chen, Ingrid L., Issam Koleilat, Krystina Choinski, John Phair, and Matthew E. Hirschtritt. 2021. "Trends in Ethnicity, Race, and Sex among Psychiatry and Non-Psychiatry Residency Applicants, 2008–2019." *Academic Psychiatry* 45 (4): 445–50.

Chodorow, Nancy. 1999. *The Power of Feelings: Personal Meaning in Psychoanalysis, Gender and Culture.* New Haven, CT: Yale University Press.

Clarke, Adele, and Joan H. Fujimura, eds. 1992. *The Right Tools for the Job: At Work in Twentieth-Century Life Sciences.* Princeton, NJ: Princeton University Press.

Collins, Harry M. 1974. "The TEA Set: Tacit Knowledge and Scientific Networks." *Science Studies* 4 (2): 165–86.

———. 2010. *Tacit and Explicit Knowledge.* Chicago: University of Chicago Press.

Collins, Harry M., and Robert Evans. 2007. *Rethinking Expertise.* Chicago: University of Chicago Press.

Coser, Rose Laub. 1961. "Insulation from Observability and Types of Social Conformity." *American Sociological Review* 26 (1): 28–39.

———. 1979. *Training in Ambiguity: Learning through Doing in a Mental Hospital.* New York: Free Press.

Craciun, Mariana. 2018. "Emotions and Knowledge in Expert Work: A Comparison of Two Psychotherapies." *American Journal of Sociology* 123 (4): 959–1003.

Cuijpers, Pim, Annemieke van Straten, Gerhard Andersson, and Patricia van Oppen. 2008. "Psychotherapy for Depression in Adults: A Meta-Analysis of Comparative Outcome Studies." *Journal of Counseling and Clinical Psychology* 76 (6): 909–22.

Cuijpers, Pim, Annemieke van Straten, Josien Schuurmans, Patricia van Oppen, Steven D. Hollon, and Gerhard Andersson. 2010. "Psychotherapy for Chronic Major Depression and Dysthymia: A Meta-Analysis." *Clinical Psychology Review* 30 (1): 51–62.

Daston, Lorraine, and Peter Galison. 1992. "The Image of Objectivity." *Representations* 40:81–128.

———. 2007. *Objectivity.* Cambridge, MA: Zone Books.

David, Daniel, Ioana Cristea, and Stefan G. Hofmann. 2018. "Why Cognitive Behavioral Therapy Is the Current Gold Standard of Psychotherapy." *Frontiers in Psychiatry* 9:4–4.

Davis, Joseph E. 2020. *Chemically Imbalanced: Everyday Suffering, Medication, and Our Troubled Quest for Self-Mastery.* Chicago: University of Chicago Press.

Davydow, Dimitry, O. Joseph Bienvenu, John Lipsey, and Karen Swartz. 2008. "Factors Influencing the Choice of a Psychiatric Residency Program: A Survey of Applicants to the Johns Hopkins Residency Program in Psychiatry." *Academic Psychiatry* 32 (2): 143–46.

de Leon, Jose. 2016. "Pharmacogenetic Tests in Psychiatry from Fear to Failure to Hype." *Journal of Clinical Psychopharmacology* 36 (4): 299–304.

DelVecchio Good, Mary-Jo. (1995) 1998. *American Medicine, the Quest for Competence.* Berkeley: University of California Press.

Detre, Thomas, and Margaret C. McDonald. 1997. "Managed Care and the Future of Psychiatry." *Archives of General Psychiatry* 54 (3): 201–4.

DiBenigno, Julia. 2018. "Anchored Personalization in Managing Goal Conflict between Professional Groups: The Case of U.S. Army Mental Health Care." *Administrative Science Quarterly* 63 (3): 526–69.

———. 2020. "Rapid Relationality: How Peripheral Experts Build a Foundation for Influence with Line Managers." *Administrative Science Quarterly* 65 (1): 20–60.

DiBenigno, Julia, and Katherine C. Kellogg. 2014. "Beyond Occupational Differences: The Importance of Crosscutting Demographics and Dyadic Toolkits for Collaboration in a U.S. Hospital." *Administrative Science Quarterly* 59 (3): 375–408.

Dobbin, Frank, and Erin L. Kelly. 2007. "How to Stop Harassment: Professional Construction of Legal Compliance in Organizations." *American Journal of Sociology* 112 (4):1203–43.

Dougherty, Darin D., Brian P. Brennan, S. Evelyn Stewart, Sabine Wilhelm, Alik S. Widge, and Scott L. Rauch. 2018. "Neuroscientifically Informed Formulation and Treatment Planning for Patients with Obsessive-Compulsive Disorder: A Review." *JAMA Psychiatry* 75 (10): 1081–87.

Douglas, Carolyn J. 2008. "Teaching Supportive Psychotherapy to Psychiatric Residents." *American Journal of Psychiatry* 165 (4): 445–52.

Douglas, Mary. 1966. *Purity and Danger: An Analysis of the Concepts of Pollution and Taboo.* New York: Routledge.

———. 1984. "The Social Preconditions of Radical Scepticism." *Sociological Review* 32 (1): 68–87.

Downey, Gregory J., Noah Weeth Feinstein, Daniel Lee Kleinman, Sigrid Peterson, and Chisato Fukuda. 2016. "The Frictions of Interdisciplinarity: The Case of the Wisconsin Institutes for Discovery." In Fricket, Albert, and Prainsack, *Investigating Interdisciplinary Collaboration*, 47–64.

Dreyfus, Hubert L., and Stuart E. Dreyfus. 2005. "Peripheral Vision: Expertise in Real World Contexts." *Organizational Studies* 26 (5): 779–92.

Dubinskas, Frank A. 1988. *Making Time: Ethnographies of High-Technology Organizations.* Philadelphia: Temple University Press.

Durkheim, Émile. (1912) 1995. *The Elementary Forms of Religious Life.* New York: Free Press.

Eisenberg, Leon. 1983. "The Subjective in Medicine." *Perspectives in Biology and Medicine* 27 (1): 48–61.

Eissler, Kurt R. 1974. "On Some Theoretical and Technical Problems Regarding the Payment of Fees for Psychoanalytic Treatment." *International Review of Psychoanalysis* 1:73–101.

Emirbayer, Mustafa. 1997. "Manifesto for a Relational Sociology." *American Journal of Sociology* 103 (2): 281–317.

Engel, George L. 1977. "The Need for a New Medical Model: A Challenge for Biomedicine." *Science* 196 (4286): 129–36.

Epstein, Steven. 1996. *Impure Science: AIDS, Activism, and the Politics of Knowledge.* Berkeley: University of California Press.

———. 1997. "Activism, Drug Regulation, and the Politics of Therapeutic Evaluation in the AIDS Era: A Case Study of DdC and the 'Surrogate Markers' Debate." *Social Studies of Science* 27 (5): 691–726.

Estroff, Sue E. 1981. *Making It Crazy: An Ethnography of Psychiatric Clients in an American Community.* Berkeley: University of California Press.

Eyal, Gil. 2006. *The Disenchantment of the Orient: Expertise in Arab Affairs and the Israeli State*. Stanford, CA: Stanford University Press.

———. 2013. "For a Sociology of Expertise: The Social Origins of the Autism Epidemic." *American Journal of Sociology* 118 (4): 863–907.

Feighner, John P., Eli Robins, Samuel B. Guze, Robert A. Woodruff Jr., George Winokur, and Rodrigo Munoz. 1972. "Diagnostic Criteria for Use in Psychiatric Research." *Archives of General Psychiatry* 26 (1): 57–63.

Fine, Gary Alan. 1990. "Organizational Time: Temporal Demands and the Experience of Work in Restaurant Kitchens." *Social Forces* 69 (1): 95–114.

———. 2019. "Relational Distance and Epistemic Generosity: The Power of Detachment in Skeptical Ethnography." *Sociological Methods and Research* 48 (4): 828–49.

Fink, Paul J. 1988. "Is "Biopsychosocial" the Psychiatric Shibboleth?" *American Journal of Psychiatry* 145 (9): 1061-7.

Flaherty, Michael G. 2002. "Making Time: Agency and the Construction of Temporal Experience." *Symbolic Interaction* 25 (3): 379–88.

Fourcade, Marion. 2009. *Economists and Societies: Discipline and Profession in the United States, Britain, and France, 1890s to 1990s*. Princeton, NJ: Princeton University Press.

Fox, Renee C. 1957. "Training for Uncertainty." In *The Student-Physician*, edited by Robert K. Merton, George Reader, and Patricia L. Kendall, 207–41. Cambridge, MA: Harvard University Press.

———. 1974. *Experiment Perilous: Physicians and Patients Facing the Unknown*. Philadelphia: University of Pennsylvania Press.

———. 1980. "The Evolution of Medical Uncertainty." *Milbank Memorial Fund Quarterly* 58 (1): 1–49.

Freedheim, Donald K. 1992. *History of Psychotherapy: A Century of Change*. Washington, DC: American Psychological Association.

Freidson, Elliott. 1970. *Profession of Medicine: A Study of Sociology of Applied Knowledge*. Chicago: University of Chicago Press.

Freud, Sigmund. 1961. *Five Lectures on Psycho-Analysis*. New York: Norton.

———. 1963. *Collected Papers*. New York: Collier Books.

Frickel, Scott, Mathieu Albert, and Barbara Prainsack, eds. 2016. *Investigating Interdisciplinary Collaboration: Theory and Practice across Disciplines*. New Brunswick, NJ: Rutgers University Press.

Fujimura, Joan H. 1987. "Constructing 'Do-Able' Problems in Cancer Research: Articulating Alignment." *Social Studies of Science* 17 (2): 257–93.

Furlong, Allannah. 1992. "Some Technical and Theoretical Considerations Regarding the Missed Session." *International Journal of Psychoanalysis* 73 (4): 701–18.

Gabbard, Glen O. 1994. "On Love and Lust in Erotic Transference." *Journal of the American Psychoanalytic Association* 42 (2): 385–86.

———. 2004. *Long-Term Psychodynamic Psychotherapy: A Basic Text*. Washington, DC: American Psychiatric Association.

———. 2007. "Psychotherapy in Psychiatry." *International Review of Psychiatry* 19 (1): 5–12.

Gabbard, Glen O., John G. Gunderson, and Peter Fonagy. 2002. "The Place of Psychoanalytic Treatments within Psychiatry." *Archives of General Psychiatry* 59 (6): 505–10.

Gabbard, Glen O., and Jerald Kay. 2001. "The Fate of Integrated Treatment: Whatever Happened to the Biopsychosocial Psychiatrist?" *American Journal of Psychiatry* 158 (12): 1956–63.

Galison, Peter. 1999. "Trading Zone: Coordinating Action and Belief." In *The Science Studies Reader,* edited by Mario Biagioli, 137–60. New York: Routledge.

Gieryn, Thomas F. 1983. "Boundary-Work and the Demarcation of Science from Non-Science—Strains and Interests in Professional Ideologies of Scientists." *American Sociological Review* 48 (6): 781–95.

———. 1999. *Cultural Boundaries of Science: Credibility on the Line.* Chicago: University of Chicago Press.

———. 2006. "City as Truth-Spot." *Social Studies of Science* 36 (1): 5–38.

Gill, Matthew. 2009. *Accountants' Truth: Knowledge and Ethics in the Financial World.* Oxford: Oxford University Press.

Giordano, Frank L., and David F. Briones. 2003. "Assessing Residents' Competence in Psychotherapy." *Academic Psychiatry* 27 (3): 145–47.

Glaeser, Andreas. 2010. *Political Epistemics: The Secret Police, the Opposition, and the End of East German Socialism.* Chicago: University of Chicago Press.

Glass, Carol R., and Diane B Arnkoff. 1992. "Behavior Therapy." In Freedheim, *History of Psychotherapy,* 687–28.

Goffman, Erving. 1959. *The Presentation of Self in Everyday Life.* Garden City, NY: Doubleday.

———. 1961. *Asylums: Essay on the Social Institution of Mental Patients and Other Inmates.* New York: First Anchor Books.

———. 1963. *Stigma: Notes on the Management of Spoiled Identity.* Englewood Cliffs, NJ: Prentice-Hall.

Goin, Marcia Kraft. 2001. "Split Treatment: The Psychotherapy Role of the Prescribing Psychiatrist." *Psychiatric Services* 52 (5): 605–6, 609.

Goldberg, Joseph F., Joshua D. Rosenblat, Roger S. McIntyre, Sheldon H. Preskorn, and Jose de Leon. 2019. "Clinical versus Statistical Significance of Pharmacogenomic-Guided Antidepressant Therapy: What's Really Being Measured and Marketed?" Letter to the editor. *Journal of Psychiatric Research* 114:208–9.

Goldstein, William N. 2000. "The Transference in Psychotherapy." *American Journal of Psychotherapy* 54 (2): 167–71.

Good, Byron. 1994. *Medicine, Rationality, and Experience: An Anthropological Perspective.* Cambridge: Cambridge University Press.

Goodwin, Charles. 1994. "Professional Vision." *American Anthropologist* 96 (3): 606–33.

Gorman, Elizabeth H., and Rebecca L. Sandefur. 2011. "'Golden Age,' Quiescence, and Revival: How the Sociology of Professions Became the Study of Knowledge-Based Work." *Work and Occupations* 38 (3): 275–302.

Greenhalgh, Joanne, Rob Flynn, Andrew F. Long, and Sarah Tyson. 2008. "Tacit and Encoded Knowledge in the Use of Standardised Outcome Measures in Multidisciplinary Team Decision Making: A Case Study of in-Patient Neurorehabilitation." *Social Science & Medicine* 67 (1): 183–94.

Grinker, Roy R. Sr. 1964. "Psychiatry Rides Madly in All Directions." *Archives of General Psychiatry* 10 (3): 228–37.

Grob, Gerald N. 1994. *The Mad among Us: A History of the Care of America's Mentally Ill.* New York: Free Press.

Guenther, Katja. 2015. *Localization and Its Discontents: A Genealogy of Psychoanalysis and the Neuro Disciplines*. Chicago: University of Chicago Press.

Guerrero, Anthony P. S., Rashi Aggarwal, Richard Balon, Eugene V. Beresin, Mary K. Morreale, John Coverdale, Alan K. Louie, and Adam M. Brenner. 2020. "The Competency Movement in Psychiatric Education: 2020 View." *Academic Psychiatry* 44 (6): 651–53.

Guidi, Jenny, and Giovanni A. Fava. 2021. "Sequential Combination of Pharmacotherapy and Psychotherapy in Major Depressive Disorder: A Systematic Review and Meta-Analysis." *JAMA Psychiatry* 78:261–69.

Guidi, Jenny, Elena Tomba, and Giovanni A. Fava. 2016. "The Sequential Integration of Pharmacotherapy and Psychotherapy in the Treatment of Major Depressive Disorder: A Meta-Analysis of the Sequential Model and a Critical Review of the Literature." *American Journal of Psychiatry* 173 (2): 128–37.

Haak, Jennifer Lynn, and David Kaye. 2009. "Personal Psychotherapy during Residency Training: A Survey of Psychiatric Residents." *Academic Psychiatry* 33 (4): 323–26.

Haas, Jack, and William Shaffir. 1977. "The Professionalization of Medical Students: Developing Competence and a Cloak of Competence." *Symbolic Interaction* 1 (1): 71–88.

———. 1982. "Taking on the Role of Doctor: A Dramaturgical Analysis of Professionalization." *Symbolic Interaction* 5 (2): 187–203.

Haas, Peter M. 1992. "Introduction: Epistemic Communities and International Policy Coordination." *International Organization* 46 (1): 1–35.

Hadjipavlou, George, Carlos A. Hernandez, and John S. Ogrodniczuk. 2015. "Psychotherapy in Contemporary Psychiatric Practice." *Canadian Journal of Psychiatry* 60 (6): 294–300.

Hale, Nathan G. 1971. *Freud and the Americans: The Beginnings of Psychoanalysis in the United States, 1876–1917*. New York: Oxford University Press.

———. 1995. *The Rise and Crisis of Psychoanalysis in the United States: Freud and the Americans, 1917–1985*. New York: Oxford University Press.

Halpern, Sydney A. 1992. "Dynamics of Professional Control: Internal Coalitions and Crossprofessional Boundaries." *American Journal of Sociology* 97 (4): 994–1021.

Haraway, Donna J. 1988. "Situated Knowledges: The Science Question in Feminism and the Privilege of Partial Perspective." *Feminist Studies* 14 (3): 575–99.

———. 1997. *Modest-Witness@Second-Millennium.FemaleMan-Meets-OncoMouse: Feminism and Technoscience*. New York: Routledge.

Hardin, Russell. 2002. *Trust and Trustworthiness*. New York: Russell Sage Foundation.

Harrington, Anne. 2019. *Mind Fixers: Psychiatry's Troubled Search for the Biology of Mental Illness*. New York: W. W. Norton.

Hartmann, Lawrence. 1992. "Presidential Address: Reflections on Humane Values and Biopsychosocial Integration." *American Journal of Psychiatry* 149 (9): 1135–41.

Healy, David. 1997. *The Antidepressant Era*. Cambridge, MA: Harvard University Press.

———. 2002. *The Creation of Psychopharmacology*. Cambridge, MA: Harvard University Press.

Herzberg, David L. 2009. *Happy Pills in America: From Miltown to Prozac*. Baltimore, MD: Johns Hopkins University Press.

Hofmann, Stefan G., Gordon J. G. Asmundson, and Aaron T. Beck. 2013. "The Science of Cognitive Therapy." *Behavior Therapy* 44 (2): 199–212.

Holloway, Kelly. 2014. "Uneasy Subjects: Medical Students' Conflicts over the Pharmaceutical Industry." *Social Science & Medicine* 114:113–20.

Horwitz, Allan V. 2002. *Creating Mental Illness.* Chicago: University of Chicago Press.

———. 2007. "Distinguishing Distress from Disorder as Psychological Outcomes of Stressful Social Arrangements." *Health* 11 (3): 273–89.

Howes, Oliver D., Michael E. Thase, and Toby Pillinger. 2022. "Treatment Resistance in Psychiatry: State of the Art and New Directions." *Molecular Psychiatry* 27 (1): 58–72.

Hughes, Everett C. 1958. *Men and Their Work.* Chicago: Free Press.

Husarewycz, M. Natalie, William Fleisher, and Kurt Skakum. 2015. "Medical Training in Psychiatric Residency: The PGY-1 Experience, 2014 Update." *Canadian Journal of Psychiatry* 60 (6): 1–8.

Ibarra, Herminia. 1999. "Provisional Selves: Experimenting with Image and Identity in Professional Adaptation." *Administrative Science Quarterly* 44 (4): 764–91.

Ibarra, Herminia, and Otilia Obodaru. 2016. "Betwixt and between Identities: Liminal Experience in Contemporary Careers." *Research in Organizational Behavior* 36:47–64.

Insel, Thomas. 2022. *Healing: Our Path from Mental Illness to Mental Health.* New York: Penguin Press.

Jacobs, Theodore J. 1991. *The Use of the Self: Countertransference and Communication in the Analytic Situation.* Madison, CT: International Universities Press.

———. 1999. "Countertransference Past and Present: A Review of the Concept. " *International Journal of Psychoanalysis* 80:575–94.

Jenkins, Tania M. 2020. *Doctors' Orders: The Making of Status Hierarchies in an Elite Profession.* New York: Columbia University Press.

Jibson, Michael D. 2006. "Medical Education and the Pharmaceutical Industry: Managing an Uneasy Alliance." *Academic Psychiatry* 30 (1): 36–39.

Kalin, Ned H. 2022. "Spanning Treatment Modalities: Psychotherapy, Psychopharmacology, and Neuromodulation." *American Journal of Psychiatry* 179 (2): 75–78.

Kandel, Eric R. 1998. "A New Intellectual Framework for Psychiatry." *American Journal of Psychiatry* 155 (4): 457–69.

Kay, Jerald. 1996. "New Challenges to the Faculty in the Education of Psychiatrists." *Bulletin of the Menninger Clinic* 60 (3): 285.

Kay, Jerald, and Michael F. Myers. 2014. "Current State of Psychotherapy Training: Preparing for the Future." *Psychodynamic Psychiatry* 42 (3): 557–73.

Kazantzis, Nikolaos, Georgios K. Lampropoulos, and Frank P. Deane. 2005. "A National Survey of Practicing Psychologists' Use and Attitudes toward Homework in Psychotherapy." *Journal of Consulting and Clinical Psychology* 73 (4): 742–48.

Kazantzis, Nikolaos, Craig Whittington, Leah Zelencich, Michael Kyrios, Peter J. Norton, and Stefan G. Hofmann. 2016. "Quantity and Quality of Homework Compliance: A Meta-Analysis of Relations with Outcome in Cognitive Behavior Therapy." *Behavior Therapy* 47 (5): 755–72.

Kellogg, Katherine C. 2011. *Challenging Operations: Medical Reform and Resistance in Surgery.* Chicago: University of Chicago Press.

———. 2014. "Brokerage Professions and Implementing Reform in an Age of Experts." *American Sociological Review* 79 (5): 912–41.

Kellogg, Katherine C., Wanda J. Orlikowski, and JoAnne Yates. 2006. "Life in the Trading Zone: Structuring Coordination across Boundaries in Postbureaucratic Organizations." *Organization Science* 17 (1): 22–44.

Khurshid, Khurshid A., Jeffrey I. Bennett, Sandy Vicari, Karen L. Lee, and Karen E.
Broquet. 2005. "Residency Programs and Psychotherapy Competencies: A Survey
of Chief Residents." *Academic Psychiatry* 29 (5): 452–58.

Kirk, Stuart A., and Herb Kutchins. 1992. *The Selling of DSM: The Rhetoric of Science in
Psychiatry.* New York: A. de Gruyter.

Kirsch, Irving 2010. *The Emperor's New Drugs: Exploding the Antidepressant Myth.*
New York: Basic Books.

Kleinman, Arthur. 1988. *Rethinking Psychiatry: From Cultural Category to Personal
Experience.* New York: Free Press.

Klerman, Gerald L, Myrna M. Weissman, Bruce J. Rounsaville, and Eve S. Chevron.
1984. *Interpersonal Psychotherapy of Depression.* New York: Basic Books.

Klitzman, Robert. 1995. *In a House of Dreams and Glass: Becoming a Psychiatrist.*
New York: Simon & Schuster.

Knorr Cetina, Karin. 1992. "The Couch, the Cathedral, and the Laboratory: On the
Relationship between Experiment and Laboratory in Science." In *Science as Practice
and Culture,* edited by Andrew Pickering, 113–38. Chicago: University of Chicago
Press.

———. 1999. *Epistemic Cultures: How the Sciences Make Knowledge.* Cambridge, MA:
Harvard University Press.

Kovach, Jessica G., William R. Dubin, and Christopher J. Combs. 2015. "Psychotherapy Training: Residents' Perceptions and Experiences." *Academic Psychiatry* 39 (5):
567–74.

Kunda, Gideon. 1992. *Engineering Culture: Control and Commitment in a High-Tech
Corporation.* Philadelphia, PA: Temple University Press.

Lakoff, Andrew. 2005a. "Diagnostic Liquidity: Mental Illness and the Global Trade in
DNA." *Theory and Society* 34(1): 63–92.

———. 2005b. *Pharmaceutical Reason: Knowledge and Value in Global Psychiatry.*
Cambridge: Cambridge University Press.

Lamont, Michèle. 1992. *Money, Morals, and Manners: The Culture of the French and
American Upper-Middle Class.* Chicago: University of Chicago Press.

Lamont, Michèle, and Virag Molnar. 2002. "The Study of Boundaries in the Social
Sciences." *Annual Review of Sociology* 28:167–95.

Lampland, Martha, and Susan Leigh Star. 2009. *Standards and Their Stories: How
Quantifying, Classifying, and Formalizing Practices Shape Everyday Life.* Ithaca, NY:
Cornell University Press.

Lanouette, Nicole M., Christina Calabrese, Andres F. Sciolla, Robin Bitner, Geor-
gian Mustata, Jennifer Lynn Haak, Sidney Zisook, and Laura B. Dunn. 2011. "Do
Psychiatry Residents Identify as Psychotherapists? A Multisite Survey." *Annals of
Clinical Psychiatry* 23 (1): 30–39.

Latour, Bruno. 1987. *Science in Action: How to Follow Scientists and Engineers through
Society.* Cambridge, MA: Harvard University Press.

Latour, Bruno, and Steve Woolgar. 1979. *Laboratory Life: The Social Construction of
Scientific Facts.* Beverly Hills, CA: Sage.

Lave, Jean, and Etienne Wenger. 1991. *Situated Learning: Legitimate Peripheral Participation.* Cambridge: Cambridge University Press.

Leichsenring, Falk. 2005. "Are Psychodynamic and Psychoanalytic Therapies
Effective? A Review of Empirical Data." *International Journal of Psychoanalysis*
86:841–68.

————. 2009. "Psychodynamic Psychotherapy: A Review of Efficacy and Effectiveness Studies." In *Handbook of Evidence-Based Psychodynamic Psychotherapy: Bridging the Gap between Science and Practice*, edited by Raymond A. Levy and J. Stuart Ablon, 3–27. New York: Humana Press.

Leichsenring, Falk, Wolfgang Hiller, Michael Weissberg, and Eric Leibing. 2006. "Cognitive-Behavioral Therapy and Psychodynamic Psychotherapy: Techniques, Efficacy, and Indications." *American Journal of Psychotherapy* 60 (3): 233.

Leichsenring, Falk, Frank Leweke, Susanne Klein, and Christiane Steinert. 2015. "The Empirical Status of Psychodynamic Psychotherapy—An Update: Bambi's Alive and Kicking." *Psychotherapy and Psychosomatics* 84 (3):129–48.

Leichsenring, Falk, and Sven Rabung. 2008. "Effectiveness of Long-Term Psychodynamic Psychotherapy—A Meta-Analysis." *Journal of the American Medical Association* 300 (13): 1551–65.

————. 2011. "Long-Term Psychodynamic Psychotherapy in Complex Mental Disorders: Update of a Meta-Analysis." *British Journal of Psychiatry* 199 (1): 15–22.

Leichsenring, Falk, Simone Salzer, Manfred E. Beutel, Stephan Herpertz, Wolfgang Hiller, Juergen Hoyer, Johannes Huesing, Peter Joraschky, Bjoern Nolting, Karin Poehlmann, Viktoria Ritter, Ulrich Stangier, Bernhard Strauss, Nina Stuhldreher, Susan Tefikow, Tobias Teismann, Ulrike Willutzki, Joerg Wiltink, and Eric Leibing. 2013. "Psychodynamic Therapy and Cognitive-Behavioral Therapy in Social Anxiety Disorder: A Multicenter Randomized Controlled Trial." *American Journal of Psychiatry* 170 (7): 759–67.

Leichsenring, Falk, and Christiane Steinert. 2017. "Is Cognitive Behavioral Therapy the Gold Standard for Psychotherapy? The Need for Plurality in Treatment and Research." *Journal of the American Medical Association* 318 (14): 1323–24.

Leuzinger-Bohleber, Marianne, and Horst Kachele, eds. 2015. *An Open Door Review of Outcome and Process Studies in Psychoanalysis.* 3rd ed. London: International Psychoanalytical Association.

Library of Congress. 2022. "Project on the Decade of the Brain." Updated February 8, 2022. https://www.loc.gov/loc/brain/.

Lieberman, Jeffrey, and Ogi Ogas. 2015. *Shrinks: The Untold Story of Psychiatry.* New York: Little, Brown.

Light, Donald Jr. 1979. "Uncertainty and Control in Professional Training." *Journal of Health and Social Behavior* 20 (4): 310–22.

————. 1980. *Becoming Psychiatrists: The Professional Transformation of Self.* New York: Norton.

Linehan, Marsha. 1993. *Skills Training Manual for Treating Borderline Personality Disorder.* New York: Guilford Press.

Linehan, Marsha M., Erin F. Ward-Ciesielski, and Andrada D. Neacsiu. 2012. "Emerging Approaches to Counseling Intervention: Dialectical Behavior Therapy." *Counseling Psychologist* 40 (7): 1003.

Link, Bruce G., and Jo C. Phelan. 2017. "Labeling and Stigma." In *A Handbook for the Study of Mental Health: Social Contexts, Theories, and Systems*, 3rd ed., edited by Teresa Scheid and Eric Wright, 393–408. New York: Cambridge University Press.

Locke, Karen, Karen Golden-Biddle, and Martha S. Feldman. 2008. "Making Doubt Generative: Rethinking the Role of Doubt in the Research Process." *Organization Science* 19 (6): 907–18.

Luborsky, Lester, Barton Singer, and Lise Luborsky. 1975. "Comparative Studies of Psychotherapies: Is It True That 'Everyone Has Won and All Must Have Prizes'?" *Archives of General Psychiatry* 32 (8): 995–1008.

Luhrmann, Tanya M. 2000. *Of Two Minds: An Anthropologist Looks at American Psychiatry.* New York: Vintage Books.

———. 2020. *How God Becomes Real: Kindling the Presence of Invisible Others.* Princeton, NJ: Princeton University Press.

Lunbeck, Elizabeth. 1994. *The Psychiatric Persuasion: Knowledge, Gender, and Power in Modern America.* Princeton, NJ: Princeton University Press.

Lurie, Scott N. "Comments on Task Force Report on Psychiatric Residency." 1990. *American Journal of Psychiatry.* 147 (8): 1096.

Mark, Joshua. 2001. "The Challenges of Split Treatment." *Psychiatric Services* 52 (9): 1254–55.

Mark, Tami L., Katharine R. Levit, and Jeffrey A. Buck. 2009. "Psychotropic Drug Prescriptions by Medical Specialty." *Psychiatric Services* 60 (9): 1167–67.

Mark, Tami L., William Olesiuk, Mir M. Ali, Laura J. Sherman, Ryan Mutter, and Judith L. Teich. 2018. "Differential Reimbursement of Psychiatric Services by Psychiatrists and Other Medical Providers." *Psychiatric Services* 69 (3): 281–85.

Markowitz, John C., and Myrna M. Weissman. 2012. "Interpersonal Psychotherapy: Past, Present and Future." *Clinical Psychology & Psychotherapy* 19 (2): 99–105.

Maslej, Marta M., Toshiaki A. Furukawa, Andrea Cipriani, Paul W. Andrews, and Benoit H. Mulsant. 2021. "Individual Differences in Response to Antidepressants: A Meta-Analysis of Placebo-Controlled Randomized Clinical Trials." *JAMA Psychiatry* 78 (5): 490–97.

McGlynn, Elizabeth A., Steven M. Asch, John Adams, Joan Keesey, Jennifer Hicks, Alison DeCristofaro, and Eve A. Kerr. 2003. "The Quality of Health Care Delivered to Adults in the United States." *New England Journal of Medicine* 348 (26): 2635–45.

Mechanic, David. 1998. "Emerging Trends in Mental Health Policy and Practice. " *Health Affairs* 17 (6): 82–98.

———. 2008. *Mental Health and Social Policy: Beyond Managed Care.* Boston: Pearson/ Allyn and Bacon.

Medina, José. 2013. *The Epistemology of Resistance: Gender and Racial Oppression, Epistemic Injustice, and Resistant Imaginations.* New York: Oxford University Press.

Mellman, Lisa A. 2006. "How Endangered Is Dynamic Psychiatry in Residency Training?" *Journal of the American Academy of Psychoanalysis and Dynamic Psychiatry* 34 (1): 127–33.

Mellman, Lisa A., and Eugene Beresin. 2003. "Psychotherapy Competencies: Development and Implementation." *Academic Psychiatry* 27 (3): 149–53.

Menchik, Daniel A. 2020. "Moving from Adoption to Use: Physicians' Mixed Commitments in Deciding to Use Robotic Technologies." *Work and Occupations* 47 (3): 314–47.

Merton, Robert King. 1973. *The Sociology of Science: Theoretical and Empirical Investigations.* Chicago: University of Chicago Press.

Merton, Robert King, and Elinor G. Barber. (1963) 1976. "Sociological Ambivalence." In *Sociological Ambivalence and Other Essays,* edited by Robert K. Merton, 3–31. New York: Free Press.

Merton, Robert King, George E. Reader, and Patricia Kendall, eds. 1957. *The Student-Physician: Introductory Studies in the Sociology of Medical Education.* Cambridge, MA: Harvard University Press.

Mertz, Elizabeth. 2007. *The Language of Law School: Learning to "Think like a Lawyer."* New York: Oxford University Press.

Metzl, Jonathan. 2003. *Prozac on the Couch: Prescribing Gender in the Era of Wonder Drugs.* Durham, NC: Duke University Press.

Miller, Sheldon I., James H. Scully Jr., and Daniel K. Winstead. 2003. "The Evolution of Core Competencies in Psychiatry." *Academic Psychiatry* 27 (3): 128–30.

Mintz, David. 2019. "The Caucus on Psychotherapy: A Voice for Psychotherapy at APA." *Psychiatric News* (online edition), July 25, 2019. https://doi.org/10.1176/appi.pn.2019.8a19.

Mitchell, Stephen A., and Margaret J. Black. 1995. *Freud and Beyond: A History of Modern Psychoanalytic Thought.* New York: Basic Books.

Mizrachi, Nissim, and Judith T. Shuval. 2005. "Between Formal and Enacted Policy: Changing the Contours of Boundaries." *Social Science & Medicine* 60 (7): 1649–60.

Moffic, H. Steven. 1990. "Comments on Task Force Report on Psychiatric Residency." *American Journal of Psychiatry* 147 (8): 1097.

Mohl, Paul C. 2004. "Assessing Psychotherapy Competence." *Academic Psychiatry* 28 (3): 251–53.

Mohl, Paul C., James Lomax, Allan Tasman, Carlyle Chan, William Sledge, Paul Summergrad, and Malkah Notman. 1990. "Psychotherapy Training for the Psychiatrist of the Future." *American Journal of Psychiatry* 147 (1): 7–13.

Mohl, Paul C., James W. Lomax, Allan Tasman, Carlyle H. Chan, and Paul Summergrad. 1990. "Response to Comments on Task Force Report on Psychiatric Residency." *American Journal of Psychiatry* 147 (8): 1098–98.

Moran, Mark. 2023. "Psychiatry Match Numbers Increase for 12th Consecutive Year." *Psychiatric News* (online edition), March 30, 2023. https://doi.org/10.1176/appi.pn.2023.05.5.043.

Morrissette, Matthew, and William Fleisher. 2021. "Some Essential Steps for Keeping Psychotherapy at the Core of Psychiatry Training: A Response to Belcher." *Academic Psychiatry* 45 (4): 491–93.

Morrissette, Matthew, William Fleisher, Polina Anang, and Michael Harrington. 2020. "Developing the Competent Psychiatric Psychotherapist: A Single-Site, Retrospective Study." *Counselling and Psychotherapy Research* 20 (4): 725–31.

Mullen, Linda S., Ronald O. Rieder, Robert A. Glick, Bruce Luber, and Paul J. Rosen. 2004. "Testing Psychodynamic Psychotherapy Skills among Psychiatric Residents: The Psychodynamic Psychotherapy Competency Test." *American Journal of Psychiatry* 161 (9): 1658–64.

National Institute of Mental Health (NIMH). 2022. "Mental Health Medications." Last reviewed June 2022. https://www.nimh.nih.gov/health/topics/mental-health-medications.

National Resident Matching Program. 2023. "Intro to the Match." Accessed July 10, 2023. https://www.nrmp.org/intro-to-the-match/.

Navon, Daniel 2019. *Mobilizing Mutations: Human Genetics in the Age of Patient Advocacy.* Chicago: University of Chicago Press.

Navon, Daniel, and Gil Eyal. 2016. "Looping Genomes: Diagnostic Change and the Genetic Makeup of the Autism Population." *American Journal of Sociology* 121 (5): 1416–71.

Ogden, Thomas H. 1992. "Comments on Transference and Countertransference in the Initial Analytic Meeting." *Psychoanalytic Inquiry* 12 (2): 225–47.

Orr, Douglass W. 1954. "Transference and Countertransference: A Historical Survey." *Journal of the American Psychoanalytic Association* 2 (4): 621–70.

Owen-Smith, Jason. 2001. "Managing Laboratory Work through Skepticism: Processes of Evaluation and Control." *American Sociological Review* 66 (3): 427–52.

Pachucki, Mark A., Sabrina Pendergrass, and Michele Lamont. 2007. "Boundary Processes: Recent Theoretical Developments and New Contributions." *Poetics* 35:331–51.

Panofsky, Aaron L. 2010. "A Critical Reconsideration of the Ethos and Autonomy of Science." In *Robert K. Merton: Sociology of Science and Sociology as Science*, edited by Craig Calhoun, 140–63. New York: Columbia University Press.

Parker, Gordon B., and Rebecca K. Graham. 2015. "Determinants of Treatment-Resistant Depression: The Salience of Benzodiazepines." *Journal of Nervous and Mental Disease* 203 (9): 659–63.

Parker, Gordon B., Gin S. Malhi, John G. Crawford, and Michael E. Thase. 2005. "Identifying 'Paradigm Failures' Contributing to Treatment-Resistant Depression." *Journal of Affective Disorders* 87 (2): 185–91.

Parker, John N., and Edward J. Hackett. 2012. "Hot Spots and Hot Moments in Scientific Collaborations and Social Movements." *American Sociological Review* 77 (1): 21–44.

Parloff, Morris B., and Irene Elkin. 1992. "The NIMH Treatment of Depression Collaborative Research Program." In Freedheim, *History of Psychotherapy*, 442–50.

Peirce, Charles Sanders. 1991. "The Fixation of Belief." In *Peirce on Signs: Writings on Semiotic by Charles Sanders Peirce*, edited by James Hoopes, 144–59. Durham, NC: University of North Carolina Press.

Pescosolido, Bernice A., and Jack K. Martin. 2015. "The Stigma Complex. " *Annual Review of Sociology* 41 (1): 87–116.

Pickersgill, Martyn. 2019. "Access, Accountability, and the Proliferation of Psychological Therapy: On the Introduction of the IAPT Initiative and the Transformation of Mental Healthcare." *Social Studies of Science* 49 (4): 627–50.

Pickren, Wade E., and Stanley F. Schneider, eds. 2005. *Psychology and the National Institute of Mental Health: A Historical Analysis of Science, Practice, and Policy*. Washington, DC: American Psychological Association.

Pilgrim, David. 2011. "The Hegemony of Cognitive-Behaviour Therapy in Modern Mental Health Care." *Health Sociology Review* 20 (2): 120–32.

Polanyi, Michael. (1958) 1962. *Personal Knowledge: Towards a Post-Critical Philosophy*. London: Routledge and Kegan Paul.

Porter, Theodore M. 1995. *Trust in Numbers: The Pursuit of Objectivity in Science and Public Life*. Princeton, NJ: Princeton University Press.

Pratt, Michael G., Kevin W. Rockmann, and Jeffrey B. Kaufmann. 2006. "Constructing Professional Identity: The Role of Work and Identity Learning Cycles in the Customization of Identity among Medical Residents." *Academy of Management Journal* 49 (2): 235–62.

Prentice, Rachel. 2013. *Bodies in Formation: An Ethnography of Anatomy and Surgery Education*. Durham, NC: Duke University Press.

Prochaska, James O., and John C. Norcross, eds. 2013. *Systems of Psychotherapy. A Transtheoretical Analysis*. 8th ed. Stamford, CT: Cengage Learning.

Ramírez-i-Ollé, Meritxell. 2018. "'Civil Skepticism' and the Social Construction of Knowledge: A Case in Dendroclimatology." *Social Studies of Science* 48 (6): 821–45.

Reiser, Morton F. 1988. "Are Psychiatric Educators 'Losing the Mind'?" *American Journal of Psychiatry* 145 (2): 148–53.

Rim, James I., Deborah L. Cabaniss, and David Topor. 2020. "Psychotherapy Tracks in US General Psychiatry Residency Programs: A Proxy for Trends in Psychotherapy Education?" *Academic Psychiatry* 44 (4): 423–26.

Rose-Greenland, Fiona. 2013. "Seeing the Unseen: Prospective Loading and Knowledge Forms in Archaeological Discovery." *Qualitative Sociology* 36 (3): 251–77.

Rosner, Rachael I. 2012. "Aaron T. Beck's Drawings and the Psychoanalytic Origin Story of Cognitive Therapy." *History of Psychology* 15 (1): 1–18.

———. 2014. "The Splendid Isolation of Aaron T. Beck." *Isis* 105 (4):734–58.

———. 2018. "Manualizing Psychotherapy: Aaron T. Beck and the Origins of Cognitive Therapy of Depression." *European Journal of Psychotherapy & Counselling* 20 (1): 25–47.

Roth, Julius A. 1963. *Timetables: Structuring the Passage of Time in Hospital Treatment and Other Careers*. Indianapolis, IN: Bobbs-Merrill.

Roudinesco, Elisabeth. 1990. *Jacques Lacan & Co.: A History of Psychoanalysis in France, 1925–1985*. Chicago: University of Chicago Press.

———. 2016. *Freud in His Time and Ours*. Cambridge, MA: Harvard University Press.

Sadowsky, Jonathan. 2006. "Beyond the Metaphor of the Pendulum: Electroconvulsive Therapy, Psychoanalysis, and the Styles of American Psychiatry." *Journal of the History of Medicine and Allied Sciences* 61 (1): 1–25.

———. 2021. *The Empire of Depression: A New History*. Medford, MA: Polity.

Sanacora, Gerard. 2020. "Is This Where We Stand after Decades of Research to Develop More Personalized Treatments for Depression?" *JAMA Psychiatry* 77 (6): 560–62.

Saul, Leon J. 1962. "The Erotic Transference." *Psychoanalytic Quarterly* 31 (1): 54–61.

Schechter, Kate. 2014. *Illusions of a Future: Psychoanalysis and the Biopolitics of Desire*. Durham, NC: Duke University Press.

Schnittker, Jason. 2017. *The Diagnostic System: Why the Classification of Psychiatric Disorders Is Necessary, Difficult, and Never Settled*. New York: Columbia University Press.

Schwartz, Barry. 1974. "Waiting, Exchange, and Power: The Distribution of Time in Social Systems." *American Journal of Sociology* 79 (4): 841–70.

Seron, Carroll, and Susan S. Silbey. 2009. "The Dialectic between Expert Knowledge and Professional Discretion: Accreditation, Social Control and the Limits of Instrumental Logic." *Engineering Studies* 1 (2): 101–27.

Shader, Richard I. 2015. "Some Thoughts about Medical Caring." *Journal of Clinical Psychopharmacology* 35 (2): 115–16.

Shapin, Steven. 1984. "Pump and Circumstance: Robert Boyle's Literary Technology." *Social Studies of Science* 14 (4): 481–520.

———.1994. *A Social History of Truth: Civility and Science in Seventeenth-Century England*. Chicago: University of Chicago Press.

———. 1995. "Cordelia's Love: Credibility and the Social Studies of Science." *Perspectives on Science* 3 (3): 255–75.

Shapin, Steven, and Simon Schaffer. 1985. *Leviathan and the Air-Pump: Hobbes, Boyle, and the Experimental Life*. Princeton, NJ: Princeton University Press.

Shedler, Jonathan. 2010. "The Efficacy of Psychodynamic Psychotherapy." *American Psychologist* 65 (2): 98–109.

Sher, Gila. 2016. *Epistemic Friction: An Essay on Knowledge, Truth, and Logic.* Oxford: Oxford University Press.

Silverman, Daniel, Nanette Gartrell, Mark Aronson, Michael Steer, and Susan Edbril. 1983. "In Search of the Biopsychosocial Perspective: An Experiment with Beginning Medical Students." *American Journal of Psychiatry* 140 (9): 1154–59.

Small, Mario. 2009. "How Many Cases Do I Need? On Science and the Logic of Case Selection in Field-Based Research." *Ethnography* 10 (1): 5–38.

Smilde, David. 2007. *Reason to Believe: Cultural Agency in Latin American Evangelicalism.* Berkeley: University of California Press.

Smith, Dena T. 2019. *Medicine over Mind: Mental Health Practice in the Biomedical Era.* New Brunswick, NJ: Rutgers University Press.

Smith, Mary L., and Gene V. Glass. 1977. "Meta-Analysis of Psychotherapy Outcome Studies." *American Psychologist* 32 (9): 752–60.

Smith-Doerr, Laurel, Sharla Alegria, Kaye Husbands Fealing, Debra Fitzpatrick, and Donald Tomaskovic-Devey. 2019. "Gender Pay Gaps in U.S. Federal Science Agencies: An Organizational Approach." *American Journal of Sociology* 125 (2): 534–76.

Somers, Margaret R., and Gloria D. Gibson. 1994. "Reclaiming the Epistemological 'Other': Narrative and the Social Constitution of Identity." In *Social Theory and the Politics of Identity*, edited by Craig Calhoun, 37–99. Cambridge, MA: Blackwell.

Stark, Luke. 2017. "Albert Ellis, Rational Therapy and the Media of 'Modern' Emotional Management." *History of the Human Sciences* 30 (4): 54–74.

Starr, Paul. 1982. *The Social Transformation of American Medicine.* New York: Basic Books.

Stefana, Alberto. 2017. "Erotic Transference." *British Journal of Psychotherapy* 33 (4): 505–13.

Steinert, Christiane, Thomas Munder, Sven Rabung, Jürgen Hoyer, and Falk Leichsenring. 2017. "Psychodynamic Therapy: As Efficacious as Other Empirically Supported Treatments? A Meta-Analysis Testing Equivalence of Outcomes." *American Journal of Psychiatry* 174 (10): 943–53.

Stengers, Isabelle. 1997. *Power and Invention.* Minneapolis: University of Minnesota Press.

Stevens, Rosemary. 1989. *In Sickness and in Wealth: American Hospitals in the Twentieth Century.* New York: Basic Books.

Stivers, Tanya, and Stefan Timmermans. 2020. "Medical Authority under Siege: How Clinicians Transform Patient Resistance into Acceptance." *Journal of Health and Social Behavior* 61 (1): 60–78.

Strauss, Anselm L., Leonard Schatzman, Rue Bucher, Danuta Ehrlich, and Melvin Sabschin. 1964. *Psychiatric Ideologies and Institutions.* New York: Free Press of Glencoe.

Sulloway, Frank J. 1992. *Freud, Biologist of the Mind: Beyond the Psychoanalytic Legend.* Cambridge, MA: Harvard University Press.

Swick, Susan, Sarah Hall, and Eugene Beresin. 2006. "Assessing the ACGME Competencies in Psychiatry Training Programs." *Academic Psychiatry* 30 (4): 330–51.

Swidler, Ann. 1986. "Culture in Action: Symbols and Strategies." *American Sociological Review* 51 (2): 273–86.

Swing, Susan R. 2007. "The ACGME Outcome Project: Retrospective and Prospective." *Medical Teacher* 29:648–54.

Szymczak, Julia E., and Charles L. Bosk. 2012. "Training for Efficiency: Work, Time, and Systems-Based Practice in Medical Residency." *Journal of Health and Social Behavior* 53 (3): 344–58.

Tadmon, Daniel, and Mark Olfson. 2022. "Trends in Outpatient Psychotherapy Provision by U.S. Psychiatrists: 1996–2016." *American Journal of Psychiatry* 179 (2): 110–21.

Terlizzi, Emily P., and Tina Norris. 2021. "Mental Health Treatment among Adults: United States, 2020." *NCHS Data Brief* no. 419. October 2021. https://www.cdc.gov/nchs/products/databriefs/db419.htm.

Timmermans, Stefan. 2005. "Suicide Determination and the Professional Authority of Medical Examiners." *American Sociological Review* 70 (2): 311–33.

———. 2006. *Postmortem: How Medical Examiners Explain Suspicious Deaths.* Chicago: University of Chicago Press.

Timmermans, Stefan, and Alison Angell. 2001. "Evidence-Based Medicine, Clinical Uncertainty, and Learning to Doctor." *Journal of Health and Social Behavior* 42 (4): 342–59.

Timmermans, Stefan, and Marc Berg. 2003. *The Gold Standard: The Challenge of Evidence-Based Medicine and Standardization in Health Care.* Philadelphia, PA: Temple University Press.

Tsing, Anna Lowenhaupt. 2005. *Friction: An Ethnography of Global Connection.* Princeton, NJ: Princeton University Press.

Turner, Victor Witter. 1969. *The Ritual Process: Structure and Anti-Structure.* Chicago: Aldine.

Underman, Kelly. 2020. *Feeling Medicine: How the Pelvic Exam Shapes Medical Training.* New York: NYU Press.

Underman, Kelly, and Laura E. Hirshfield. 2016. "Detached Concern? Emotional Socialization in Twenty-First Century Medical Education." *Social Science & Medicine* 160:94–101.

US Food and Drug Administration (FDA). 2014. "Selective Serotonin Reuptake Inhibitors (SSRIs) Information." Published December 23, 2014. https://www.fda.gov/drugs/information-drug-class/selective-serotonin-reuptake-inhibitors-ssris-information.

Vallas, Steven Peter. 2001. "Symbolic Boundaries and the New Division of Labor: Engineers, Workers and the Restructuring of Factory Life." *Research in Social Stratification and Mobility* 18:3–37.

van Dis, Eva A. M., Suzanne C. van Veen, Muriel A. Hagenaars, Neeltje M. Batelaan, Claudi L. H. Bockting, Rinske M. van den Heuvel, Pim Cuijpers, and Iris M. Engelhard. 2020. "Long-Term Outcomes of Cognitive Behavioral Therapy for Anxiety-Related Disorders: A Systematic Review and Meta-Analysis." *JAMA Psychiatry* 77 (3): 265–73.

van Gennep, Arnold 1960. *The Rites of Passage.* Chicago: University of Chicago Press.

Van Maanen, John. 1973. "Observations on the Making of Policemen." *Human Organization* 32 (4): 407–18.

———. 1975. "Police Socialization: A Longitudinal Examination of Job Attitudes in an Urban Police Department." *Administrative Science Quarterly* 20 (2): 207–28.

Van Maanen, John, and Stephen R. Barley. 1984. "Occupational Communities: Culture and Control in Organizations." *Research in Organizational Behavior* 6:287–365.

Vasile, Russell G., Jacqueline A. Samson, Jules Bemporad, Kerry L. Bloomingdale, David Creasey, Brenda T. Fenton, Jon E. Gudeman, and Joseph J. Schildkraut. 1987. "A Biopsychosocial Approach to Treating Patients with Affective Disorders." *American Journal of Psychiatry* 144 (3): 341–44.

Vinson, Alexandra H., and Kelly Underman. 2020. "Clinical Empathy as Emotional Labor in Medical Work." *Social Science & Medicine* 251:112904. https://doi.org/10.1016/j.socscimed.2020.112904.

Virani, Sanya, Souparno Mitra, M. Alejandra Grullón, Ayesha Khan, Jessica Kovach, and Robert O. Cotes. 2021. "International Medical Graduate Resident Physicians in Psychiatry: Decreasing Numbers, Geographic Variation, Community Correlations, and Implications." *Academic Psychiatry* 45 (1): 7–12.

Wampold, Bruce 2015. "How Important Are the Common Factors in Psychotherapy? An Update." *World Psychiatry* 14 (3): 270–77.

Waters, Mary C. 1990. *Ethnic Options: Choosing Identities in America.* Berkley: University of California Press.

———. 1994. "Ethnic and Racial Identities of Second-Generation Black Immigrants in New York City." *International Migration Review* 28 (4): 795.

———. 1999. *Black Identities: West Indian Immigrant Dreams and American Realities.* New York: Russell Sage Foundation.

Waters, Mary C., and Tomás R. Jiménez. 2005. "Assessing Immigrant Assimilation: New Empirical and Theoretical Challenges." *Annual Review of Sociology* 31:105.

Weick, Karl E., Kathleen M. Sutcliffe, and David Obstfeld. 2005. "Organizing and the Process of Sensemaking." *Organization Science* 16 (4): 409–21.

Weinrach, Stephen G. 1988. "Cognitive Therapist: A Dialogue with Aaron Beck." *Journal of Counseling & Development* 67 (3): 159.

Weishaar, Marjorie E. 1993. *Aaron T. Beck.* Thousand Oaks, CA: Sage.

Weissman, Myrna M., John C. Markowitz, and Gerald L. Klerman. 2000. *Comprehensive Guide to Interpersonal Psychotherapy.* New York: Basic Books.

West, Joyce C., Joshua E. Wilk, Donald S. Rae, William E. Narrow, and Darrel A. Regier. 2003. "Economic Grand Rounds: Financial Disincentives for the Provision of Psychotherapy." *Psychiatric Services* 54 (12): 1582–88.

Whooley, Owen. 2010. "Diagnostic Ambivalence: Psychiatric Workarounds and the Diagnostic and Statistical Manual of Mental Disorders." *Sociology of Health and Illness* 32 (3): 452–69.

———. 2013. *Knowledge in the Time of Cholera: The Struggle over American Medicine in the Nineteenth Century.* Chicago: University of Chicago Press.

———. 2014. "Nosological Reflections: The Failure of DSM-5, the Emergence of RDoC, and the Decontextualization of Mental Distress." *Society and Mental Health* 4 (2): 92–110.

———. 2016. "Measuring Mental Disorders: The Failed Commensuration Project of DSM-5." *Social Science & Medicine* 166:33–40.

———. 2019. *On the Heels of Ignorance: Psychiatry and the Politics of Not Knowing.* Chicago: University of Chicago Press.

Wilk, Joshua E., Joyce C. West, Donald S. Rae, and Darrel A. Regier. 2006. "Patterns of Adult Psychotherapy in Psychiatric Practice." *Psychiatric Services* 57 (4): 472–76.

Winfield, Taylor Paige. 2022. "Interpellative Styles: Choreographies of Identity Disruptions and Repairs." *Sociological Theory* 40 (4): 342–65.

Yager, Joel, and David Bienenfeld. 2003. "How Competent Are We to Assess Psychotherapeutic Competence in Psychiatric Residents?" *Academic Psychiatry* 27 (3): 174–81.

Yager, Joel, Jerald Kay, and Lisa Mellman. 2003. "Assessing Psychotherapy Competence: A Beginning." *Academic Psychiatry* 27 (3): 125–27.

Yager, Joel, Lisa Mellman, Eugene Rubin, and Allan Tasman. 2005. "The RRC Mandate for Residency Programs to Demonstrate Psychodynamic Psychotherapy Competency among Residents: A Debate." *Academic Psychiatry* 29 (4): 339–49.

Zerubavel, Eviatar. 1979. *Patterns of Time in Hospital Life: A Sociological Perspective.* Chicago: University of Chicago Press.

———. 1982. "The Standardization of Time: A Sociohistorical Perspective." *American Journal of Sociology* 88 (1): 1–23.

Zisook, Sidney, John R. McQuaid, Andres Sciolla, Nicole Lanouette, Christina Calabrese, and Laura B. Dunn. 2011. "Psychiatric Residents' Interest in Psychotherapy and Training Stage: A Multi-Site Survey." *American Journal of Psychotherapy* 65 (1): 47–59.

INDEX

Abbott, Andrew, 13, 177, 200n68, 206n9
Accreditation Council for Graduate Medical Education (ACGME), 7–9, 14, 22, 26, 170, 202n6, 203n23; Residency Review Committee, 7–8, 198n40
affective skills, 74–80, 89, 127, 206n8. *See also* doctor-patient relationships; empathy
American Board of Psychiatry and Neurology (ABPN), 7, 197n36. *See also* board certification
American Psychiatric Association, 1, 5, 7, 25, 174, 213n32; Committee on Psychotherapy by Psychiatrists, 197n25
American Psychological Association, 213n32
Anspach, Renee, 141, 205n4
antidepressants, 33, 114, 197n31, 208n10. *See also* SSRIs
antipsychotics, 33
anxiety: CBT treatment, 47–50, 83–84, 89, 96–100, 115, 145–46; generalized anxiety disorder, 93, 114, 207n1; medications for, 33, 208n12; psychodynamic psychotherapy and, 123–24, 153–61. *See also* benzodiazepines; exposure and response prevention; Generalized Anxiety Disorders questionnaire; mood disorders; SSRIs
apprenticeship, 20, 70, 91, 94, 171, 205nn3–4. *See also* observation; witnessing
authority: classification and, 67, 205n18; in doctor-patient relationships, 121; epistemic, 46, 53–59, 68, 204n4;

novicehood and, 61 (*see also* novicehood); as pharmacologists, 17, 36, 58, 199n56, 211n4; of supervisors, 63–64

Barber, Elinor, 14–15
Beck, Aaron, 10–11, 199n61, 199n63, 206n13
Beck, Judith, 80, 152, 206n13, 209n1
Beck Depression Inventory, 11, 47
Beck Institute, 206n13
behaviorism, 11, 86–87. *See also* CBT
benzodiazepines, 161, 208n12. *See also* anxiety; psychiatric medications
Beresin, Jeremy, 6
Bergmann, Jorg R., 204n7
biopsychiatry (biological psychiatry): competence in, 9; connections to psychotherapy, 37, 81–82, 92; as dominant framework, 25; effectiveness of, 1–3, 196n16; expertise in, 199n56; goals of, 51; history of, 4–6; limits of, 44, 69–70, 173; professional socialization in, 66–68, 118, 166, 168, 172–74; residency training, 23, 42–43. *See also* brain; neurobiology; pharmacology; psychiatric medications; psychiatry
biopsychosocial approach, 178–79, 212n27
board certification, 26, 170, 197n36, 200n69. *See also* American Board of Psychiatry and Neurology
borderline personality disorder, 2, 35, 195n10
Bosk, Charles, 210n12